THE THERAPIST'S JOURNEY

Also by Robert Taibbi

Doing Couple Therapy:
Craft and Creativity in Work with Intimate Partners,
Second Edition

Doing Family Therapy:
Craft and Creativity in Clinical Practice,
Fourth Edition

THE THERAPIST'S JOURNEY

From Meeting Your First Client to Finding Your Life's Work

ROBERT TAIBBI

THE GUILFORD PRESS
New York London

A Division of Guilford Publications, Inc.
370 Seventh Avenue, Suite 1200, New York, NY 10001
www.guilford.com

Printed in the United States of America

This book is printed on acid-free paper.

Last digit is print number: 9 8 7 6 5 4 3 2 1

Library of Congress Cataloging-in-Publication Data

Names: Taibbi, Robert, author.
Title: The therapist's journey : changes, challenges, and the art of caring / Robert Taibbi.
Description: New York, NY : The Guilford Press, [2023] | Includes bibliographical references and index.
Identifiers: LCCN 2022057839 | ISBN 9781462552412 (paperback) | ISBN 9781462552429 (cloth)
Subjects: LCSH: Self-actualization (Psychology) | Psychotherapy. | Anxiety—Prevention.
Classification: LCC BF637.S4 T33 2023 | DDC 158.1—dc23/eng/20230407
LC record available at *https://lccn.loc.gov/2022057839*

About the Author

Robert Taibbi, LCSW, is an experienced clinician, supervisor, and clinical director who has been practicing almost 50 years. He is the author of numerous books, including *Doing Family Therapy, Fourth Edition,* and *Doing Couple Therapy, Second Edition,* as well as over 300 magazine and journal articles, and writes a column titled "Fixing Families" for *Psychology Today* online. Mr. Taibbi provides training both nationally and internationally in couple therapy, family therapy, brief therapy, and clinical supervision. He has a private practice in Charlottesville, Virginia.

Acknowledgments

I'd like to thank Jim Nageotte and Jane Keislar, my editors at The Guilford Press, for their support not only on this project, but on all our previous projects over the 25-plus years we've been working together.

As I've tried to say throughout this book, our work shapes us, and what shapes the work are those we work with. As I look back over the years and the thousands of clients I have humbly tried to help, I am grateful to all of them for trusting me with their stories, teaching me their hard-earned lessons, and inspiring me with their resilience. I am also appreciative of all those readers and students who have taken the time to let me know that in some way my words have made a difference.

Finally, I want to thank my family for always cheering me on and especially my wife, Susan, for her unfailing support.

Contents

THE THERAPIST'S JOURNEY

Introduction

If you have ever taken a trip to a new and especially foreign destination, you were likely excited but also a bit anxious. You found that a good guidebook or website can be helpful by preparing you for the journey ahead. You have a map to help you get the lay of the land. There's information about all those practical things you need to know—the money and transportation systems, how to get from the airport to your hotel, what to wear, what to do when emergencies arise—when you don't feel well or are stranded—so you can make the best use of your time in this new place and not feel so overwhelmed.

And once you finally arrive and are settled in, you can sit back and read about what to expect from this new place you are suddenly in—the customs and culture of the people, what to see and do, what to avoid. Armed with this essential information, it's time to break out—find exciting day trips off the beaten path to make your journey truly your own.

This is what you may be doing now, beginning your own exciting journey into a new chapter of your life, a new profession, or a new way of being in the world. You may be at those early planning stages, just honing in on where you want to go or not yet having a clear idea of what you ultimately want to do. Or you may be further along—already landed and settled—but are unsure where to go day by day, how to make the best use of your time, how to match the place with your passions, how to handle those emergencies that might arise, how to feel less out of place, less the stranger in a strange land and more the one who has found a new home.

I wrote this book as a guide to the clinical life wherever you are starting from. The goal is to help you feel a bit less overwhelmed or unsure about how to start; to provide some basic but also some not-so-basic information so that you don't feel quite so disoriented on a bad day; to help you not only know how to handle those emergencies, but also to understand what is normal and common, so you are not fraught with anxiety and can professionally and emotionally hit the ground running so that your journey becomes the one you envisioned way back when. To do this you need to be proactive and take control of your life, go after what you want and need, and do what you have to do.

In other words, the goal is to help you feel more grounded, to help you see what you might overlook or need to appreciate, to navigate the unexpected, to look beyond this one day to imagine the many days to come.

Welcome to your journey.

About This Book

One of my goals is to create a reading environment that feels more like a conversation than a presentation. To do that I've used a mix of pronouns throughout, an informal writing style, and a number of clinical examples that are fictional and composite clients drawn from my experience. Finally, you'll find questions at the end of many chapters. They are invitations for you to reflect on your clinical skills, on your career, and on the ways your values and personality may impact your work. I hope you'll pause and consider them.

PART I

STARTING OUT

Before starting any journey, you want to start out knowing not only where you are going and what's ahead, but why you are going at all. In this part, we explore some of those questions.

CHAPTER 1

Why Do You Want to Be a Therapist?

A Question and Answer in Two Parts

No doubt you've been asked this question many times: when applying to grad school, by parents who always thought that working in engineering or IT was a secure way to go, when interviewing for a job—and undoubtedly, you've come up with some lines, some story. But when you think hard about it, you realize that those stories were maybe only half right: They were an abridged, made-for-public-consumption answer that was honest and understandable enough but geared toward moving the conversation to a different topic. Or the story was unabridged, but it had a way of changing over time as you periodically looked at yourself and your life through a new lens.

I'm challenging you to go deeper, beyond the answer you've crafted and come to feel comfortable with, and take stock once again: Why do you want to be a therapist?

Part 1: The Why

Why? Write this question down at the top of a piece of paper. Stare at it for a couple of minutes. Okay, now start writing. Write down what comes into your head without censoring, without worrying about grammar. Ask the question over and over. Keep going. If you get stuck, or think you're done, take a few deep breaths. New thought popped into your head? Great, write it down. Keep asking. . . . Okay, you've run out of steam.

Look over your list. What do you notice? Is there a theme? Surely something about helping others—but what are the variations? Is there a driving goal? A strong sense of purpose? A fantasy of accomplishment? Is there anything, now that you are truly honest with yourself, that you knew was there but was tucked away in some back closet of your mind or an experience that surprises you?

Part 2: Your Life as a Play

This is a guided imagery exercise that I've developed and used over the years. To have the best experience, you want to find a quiet space and time and not be rushed; close your eyes or look down. You can read the instructions in segments, record them with pauses, or have someone read them to you. When it's over, you can read through the debriefing to help you decode it and see what you discover.

Imagine yourself entering a theater. You walk into a lobby where many people are milling around. You walk through the lobby into the auditorium, where you take the best seat in the house. In front of you is a large stage with a curtain drawn across it.

You make yourself comfortable, and now the other people in the audience come in and take the seats around you. The house lights go dim, and the stage lights go on. A play is about to start.

The curtain rises on the first act. On stage, we see you, and you are a young child. On stage with you are one or both of your parents. Something is wrong with you—you may be crying, frightened, or worried—but something is wrong. Watch what happens, listen to what is said, see who else is there. . . .

The curtain comes down. It rises again, and we see you on stage, but now you're older, a teenager, and one or both of your parents are on the stage with you. They're talking to you about growing up: relationships and sex, careers, and education. Listen to what they say, listen to what you say back. . . .

The curtain comes down. It rises on the next act, and we see you on stage, and it is that time in your life when you are leaving home for the first time, literally moving out of the house—to go to college, to get an apartment with friends, to get married. On stage with you are one or both of your parents. Watch what happens, listen to what is said, and see if you can tell how you are feeling at the moment. . . .

The curtain comes down. It rises on the next act, and now you are a bit older, and on stage with you is someone you consider to be a mentor—it may be a college advisor, a former supervisor, or a relative—a grandparent or aunt. You are talking together and, as you do, see if you can tell what it is that you most admire about this person. . . .

The curtain comes down. It rises at a time in the present; you're at work. Watch what happens, see who is there, listen to what is said. . . .

The curtain comes down. It rises again, and the time is the far distant future, that time in your life when people see you as not only experienced but wise. And one or two people ask: Out of your years of working and living, what is it that you learned most? Listen to what you say; listen to what they say back. . . .

The play is over now. The curtain comes down, the stage lights go off, and the house lights go on. People in the audience get up and begin to leave the theater. You follow them out, and you overhear them talking about the play. Listen to what they say about it.

Okay, open your eyes. So, what did you see? The questions to ask yourself are: Of all the things you could have seen, why did you see what you did and what does it say about your life right now? What is the overall tone? What patterns run through the scenes?

Okay, let's help you debrief. Now you may have had explicit scenes or vague ones. You may have had memories instead of scenes or feelings but no clear images. That's fine. But if you did imagine something, you always want to ask yourself when doing any guided imagery exercise: Why am I imagining this now? They are like dreams—why did I dream what I did last night? It tells you something about you and your life right now. Let's walk through it. Here are some guidelines to help you interpret what you saw.

The first scene of you is as a young child with your parents. Now we could have kept this scene as a neutral one—you and your parents on stage. And out of all you could have imagined, what did you imagine: playing with your sister in the backyard, enjoying a holiday with relatives, being scolded at the dinner table? Why this image out of all possible ones? What does it say about your childhood, your life now?

But . . . we didn't do that. In this exercise, I deliberately slanted it toward the negative, that there's something wrong with you. So you see yourself sitting on the floor crying, and your mother picks you up and comforts you. Or you're crying, but she yells at you and tells you to shut up. Or your father picks you up, but you hear your mother in the background telling your father to stop babying you. Or no one pays attention to you at all.

Why is this important? Because we all leave our childhoods with an often-unconscious view of others and the world. One element of this view is trust: Is the world safe? Can I depend on others to help me when I am in need? Why is trust important to doing therapy? Because clients often have different notions of trust. For many of our clients, and even for those in our field, the answer is sadly no: The world is not safe; I need to be alert to danger; I can't depend on others; I need to take care of myself. Not only does this perception shape their expectations of you and therapy, but your expectations as well.

But the other element in this scene is those early ingrained views about helping: Is it okay for me to ask for help, to lean on others? One of your jobs as a clinician is helping others, and I would say that based on your own notions and experience, there is often a fine line between what you consider helping and . . . whining.

You as a teen—a time for what I call the "birds and the bees" talk. Most of us have never had that sit-down with our parents when they say, "Well, now that you are getting older, there're some things you should probably know." But during those teen years, we do get a lot of advice, or not, about adulthood—about work and relationships and what makes a good life. Go to college and get a job where you don't have to be like me, where you break your back or get dirty. Or don't run off to college because your friends are; instead, take some time to figure out what you really want to do. Or get married; you don't want to be alone in the world. Or don't just get married to get married. You don't want to be like me: I got married at 20 and gave away half of my adulthood. Slow down and figure out who you are before you lose yourself in a relationship. What did you hear?

What's important here is that these messages from parents often become the shoulds that run our lives. They can drive us, fill our heads and our lives, and when we don't follow them, we can feel guilty. The shoulds are different from the values we choose as an adult.

Leaving home. You are packing up your stuff, going off to college or moving to an apartment. Your dad is loading up the car; your mom is standing around a bit teary, or no, you're by yourself; no one else is around. How did you feel at the moment? Are you excited, off to a new adventure? A bit scared, unsure about what's next? A bit of both? And even if you felt excited, what were you most excited about? Not only what were you looking forward to, but what were you eager to get away from? What was that emotion?

Why is this important? In some therapy book I read somewhere a long time ago, the author said that how you felt when you left home becomes the emotional bottom line when you leave other things in your life—relationships and jobs. I don't know if this is true, but it is something to be aware of and ask yourself. When you look back on the times you left that relationship or job, is there some emotional bottom line you consistently hit—when you feel dismissed, criticized, or not appreciated or abused somehow? Now, some people never leave, they are always the "leftee," but for most of us, there is some emotional end point. Knowing it helps you understand your patterns and allows you to manage them differently and change them because, like it or not, you are likely to do many leavings at points in your life.

But there's another clinical reason for thinking about leaving home. Clients also have their own emotional bottom lines that they hit and decide it's time to go and quit. That quitting point can also be when they stop therapy. When they feel dismissed by you or criticized or not appreciated enough, they find a reason not to return. By knowing this about them early on and tracking their pattern of leaving, you know what to do and not do, how to be, and how to help them change their experience.

You and your mentor. Now some folks don't have a flesh-and-blood mentor—their mentors may be writers of books or teachers they've seen from afar. What's important is not only who your role models are, but what they do that you admire most. This tells you not only what may be missing most from your life, but can help you envision the kind of person you ultimately want to be.

The present, your job. As with all the other scenes, the underlying question is: Out of all you can see, what do you see, and what does that say about you right now? This is particularly true in this scene. Out of all you do, what is the tone of this scene—are you happy, anxious, alone, with others, feeling confident, harried? What? What does this say about the current state of you? What, if anything, do you need to do most to change the climate?

The last scene, the far-distant future. If you are going through many changes in your life right now—a breakup, in between jobs, a medical crisis—you may have difficulty seeing this scene. Your future is unclear because your present is as well. But if you did see something, what did you see? What was your answer to the question of what did you learn most through all your years of living and working? What is the moral of the story of your life? How is what you said similar to or different from what your parents or mentor said and how you wanted to be?

Finally, the audience's reaction: What did they say about the play? It was great; it was boring. The person started shakily but turned it around or seemed never to get what was wanted. These reactions are a way of stepping back and seeing our lives from a different vantage point, but what's also important is our own reaction—if they said it was boring, are you upset by that, or no, you don't care, it's your life, not theirs. How much do the opinions or imagined opinions of others shape how you see yourself and what you do?

The play is not prophecy; it is a slice of where you are in your life right now, information about you and your world of work and goals from a different part of your brain and awareness. See what you resonate with. Think about how it shapes your decision to enter this profession.

So we are back to our initial question: Why did you decide to be a therapist out of all you could be? Why this? Why now?

Mull on it and see how it applies to yourself and your work.

CHAPTER 2

Reflections

My Becoming a Therapist

My mother passed away after a relatively short run of cancer when I was twelve. I was, I am, an only child, and I didn't have a close relationship with my father. I saw him as critical, a workaholic, who, having lived through the Depression, believed that the best he could do was to "provide." In hindsight, saying I didn't handle my mother's death well is an understatement. I didn't cry before or after, though my father broke down and struggled emotionally for months. I stepped up and filled that hole in the family system—cooking and cleaning. I went from a B+ student to an A+ student because grades were important to my father. I was in the honor society, president of the ski club, did the right stuff.

But on the other side, there were signs that something was amiss. My mother died in the summer; I was out of school. I didn't tell anyone except one close friend that my mother had died; several of my friends' parents knew she had been ill, and when they asked, I said she was okay. It was only a year later, when a friend's father asked if my mother worked a lot because she never seemed to be at home, that I nonchalantly said that she had died the year before. I also started shoplifting, drinking heavily on weekends when my father started going out on dates, and even showing up to play in my band concerts drunk, unable to read the music. If you had asked how I felt about my mother's death, I would probably have shrugged and said I was okay.

Fast forward: Go to college, have the same girlfriend I met at fifteen, do well in school—Dean's List, sociology major. Married at 20 while still in school, had a son at 21. In my senior year, the university started a peer counseling program. My roommate decided to join and convinced me to do the same. The training was an alternative universe for me. Students sat in a circle on oversized pillows, emoting about all sorts of things. The training left me mystified but intrigued.

I graduated. What to do? Fortunately, my wife was working as a nurse, so we could pay the bills. But still I had a few months of panic, as I made limp applications to state jobs—probation officers and the like. I had to do something, and so I did: I applied to grad school! I was accepted into a PhD sociology program at a college in New England with a full scholarship. Good to go.

But then I met a social worker who worked with my wife at a program doing research into alcohol treatment. I had no idea what the guy did or what social work was, but he seemed like a nice guy. Hmmm . . . social work. I somehow heard about a new social work program starting in South Carolina—a good location. My wife and I were ready to get out of Dodge to someplace different. I dropped the sociology program and New England, and we headed to South Carolina. Looking back on it now, the decision seems impulsive; I stumbled into a social work program in the same way I stumbled into peer counseling in college—aware of what I was doing, but not really sure why.

When I graduated, did I have a sense that direct practice was my vocation? Not really. I had done well in placements, but felt that academic life would be . . . better, some kind of step up. I was still very much in my head. I planned to get a PhD in social work, do research, but I also realized I'd have a better chance of getting into a program if I had some experience rather than none.

So, I took a job at a family service agency right on the main street and started seeing a range of clients—families, parents, and individuals. Some of my clients looked like my parents, some looked like me. I worked with clients who talked about the abuse or loss that they not only suffered but had never shared with anyone before; clients who cried or raged. I felt overwhelmed at times, but I also got hooked.

What did I get hooked by? I'd call it controlled intimacy. My clients' experiences lingered within me, but what lingered most was that their emotional experiences lingered at all. Exposed to their emotional honesty, I too was able to reconnect with my past and get out of my head and into my emotions. Their openness to their emotional lives opened me up to my own in slow but powerful ways.

Looking back, I can see how my life was already leading me toward healing—by volunteering for the peer counseling training, by switching grad schools and programs at the last minute, by doing therapy.

These underground streams eventually came together and pushed their way to the surface of my life. Once I was hooked on working with people, and less numb from the neck down, my desire for research and academia waned.

My story is unique because it is *my* story. But it is not truly unique because I've found over the years in telling this story in my trainings that others in this profession say they have had similar experiences. Those with truly happy childhoods, as often as not, do not become therapists. Maybe we come to this place in our lives because our lives do lead us where we need to go.

Again, the question I asked in the previous chapter: Why, out of all the ways you can choose to be, did you choose this path and place in your life? Don't be surprised if your answer to that question changes over the years.

CHAPTER 3

Why Doing Therapy Is Hard Work

You're at a party where you don't know many people, so you step up and introduce yourself to a group gathered in the corner of the room. There's Sara, Henry, Martha, and Clay. Invariably the conversation turns to "And what to do you do?" Sara, it turns out, is a neurosurgeon; Henry works for himself doing custom cabinet design and building; Martha has worked forever as director of HR for a mid-size local company; and Clay is an IT guy spending most of his days troubleshooting and repairing ailing computers. Do they like their jobs? A big nod from Sara, a smaller one from Henry and Martha, and Clay gives you an "it's okay" shoulder shrug.

But then, after a couple of beats of silence, the tone shifts. "Of course, I love my job," says Sara, "but it's not nine-to-five. The stress of being on call, doing emergency surgeries at 3:00 A.M. on a Saturday when I'd rather be home in bed, or with my family." And then Henry joins in—he's fine when he's working alone in his shop, but the customers come in and can't make up their minds about what they want or change their minds midstream—drives him nuts. "Talk about midstream," pipes up Martha. "The great powers-to-be state regulators are changing policies and protocols every couple of weeks, it seems." And then Clay jumps in about how they are constantly short staffed, everybody's on fire wanting something fixed now, and he's caught between the monotony of the work and the harassment he continually feels.

"And so, what do you do? Wow, a therapist. That must be interesting . . . challenging . . . emotionally draining," and you nod your head in agreement.

Of course, you're thinking but don't say, "Yes, and it is utterly overwhelming at times because I often feel like I'm flying by the seat of my pants."

And then they smile, and you imagine them thinking, "Compared to my job, it's got to be a piece of cake. No on call, no being jerked around by the state, no hustling and being hassled all day long. All you need to do is sit there, listen, and occasionally nod your head. I could do that."

Well, I know, and you know, but they couldn't know, because even though it may not look like it from the outside, therapy is hard work. If you're having trouble articulating why it is, here's some help: what makes therapy unique and challenging.

You're Usually Working Alone and in Isolation

Sara may be in charge when she operates, but she never works alone. There are others in the room to support her practically and even emotionally. And if she wants a second opinion, another pair of hands, or backup if something goes wrong, she's likely to quickly find it. Ditto for Martha, who too works with a team. Like Sara, she may be in charge but likely has a supervisor who can tell her what changes to worry about and what to put on the back burner, who can call the state and complain to her level colleagues. Henry's a one-person show and, yes, he has to deal with customers, but most of his work is him and the wood, and the wood doesn't talk or complain much. Neither do Clay's computers and, like Sara, if he's stuck, he can probably get immediate help by going online or dialing up a tech specialist somewhere in the world.

But you, short of a client going homicidal or suicidal on the spot, got nothing. Session after session, it's just you and the client—no quick Goggle search, no backup hands or opinions unless in those rare occasions when you're doing therapy with a colleague running a group or family session. The support you get is, at best, an after-the-fact debriefing with your supervisor. It's like Sara standing by herself over the operating table.

Feeling some pressure? Maybe.

You Have to Hit the Ground Running

Sure, you worked with clients when you were doing your fieldwork or internship, but they were likely handpicked, and even if they weren't, you probably had close supervision in which you and your supervisor walked through what you could do in the upcoming sessions. But once you're on the job, the handpicking stops; with your one hour a week, you and your supervisor don't have time to mull over every case, and you no longer have a handful of cases but several handfuls. Sara, Martha, Henry, and probably even Clay developed their skills in a baby-step fashion with lots of support and a gradual increase in responsibility. For you, it's a quick zero to 60.

You Likely Have to Deal with a Wide Range of Problems

Sara doesn't do hip replacements; Henry doesn't build decks; Martha doesn't fix computers; Henry doesn't run HR. But unless you're working in a specialized setting—say, a treatment program for children on the spectrum—you're likely expected to see kids, families, adults of all ages, and all types of problems that you never encountered in your internships or past jobs. Again, it is a lot to learn, and you have to hit the ground running.

You Have High Impact and High Responsibility

If Sara wiggles her scalpel a millimeter too much to the left, she could permanently paralyze her patient. But if the wood that Henry is using splits, Clay's new memory chip isn't working, Martha's new job candidate turns up with a dirty background check, Henry grabs another piece of wood, Clay, a new chip, Martha, a new candidate—it's not the end of the world.

But in her first appointment with you, Carly says, "I've finally convinced my partner to come in with me. He's willing to come once to see if you can help us save our relationship." Or "The school says that they need to have you do an evaluation and write a letter saying that our son needs special services or they will expel him." Or "I'm really depressed; I'm at the end of my rope."

You may not be Sara, but you're certainly not like the rest. There's pressure; what you do next matters.

Your Clients Are Human, Just Like You

We're in the people business. So are the others at the party in their own ways, but not with the same intensity as you have. When Sara is doing surgery, she's likely focusing on her patient's brain and not much else. Martha, Clay, and Henry have their run-ins with their bosses and colleagues and "customers," one or two of whom may even remind them of their ex or their father or have similar tragic stories that tap into their own, but they are likely not dealing with these issues day in and day out, all day long.

This is the intimacy that makes therapy, therapy, that makes it rewarding but also draining. You're not dealing with computers or wood, résumés, or even brains, but people like you—who have the same sadness and anger and struggle with making sense of their lives as you do. That's why it's hard to turn doing therapy off at the end of the day. Clay and Henry can go back tomorrow and pick up where they left off, knowing nothing has changed. You're not so lucky, so you lie in bed at night wondering what impact your words and gestures made, whether, in the end, you really made a difference.

So, does what I've said help you explain to others and, more important, to yourself why you are in a life-changing, noble, but also challenging profession? Think about it, particularly on those days when you're apt to give yourself a hard time.

CHAPTER 4

Transitions

From the Academic to the Agency World

As we discussed in the previous chapter, your student fieldwork or internship gave you some "boots on the ground" experience, but looking back on it, you probably realize how rarefied a world it was. Just as those signs on top of cars that say "student driver" let you know you need to cut the driver some slack and lower your expectations, introducing yourself as a student to your clients probably caused them to do much the same. And as "just a student," you observed, you completed histories, probably had a few handpicked cases of your own, supplemented with plenty of close supervision to ensure you didn't do any major damage. And if you were lucky, you had one or two or even more fellow students to hang with, exchange notes, and share anxieties and woes. Those other weekdays you sat in class, engaged or bored. You had papers due in three weeks, but you could pull an all-nighter, if need be, to crank out the assignment the night before. Most of all, you probably felt antsy and anxious to wrap it up and get out.

All that changed or will change once you graduate. School friends will scatter as they go to their workplaces or back to their hometowns, and you're starting on your own as a newbie once again. The transition from "just a student" to a hard-working professional can be jarring for a lot of good reasons.

Day In, Day Out

Maybe you covered weekend shifts at Dunkin' Donuts during high school, did landscaping, or were an associate at a nonprofit during the summers in college. Or perhaps you were entrenched in something more solid—a former life in banking where you had a title and career until you decided it no longer fit who you were or wanted to be, and you took the risk to break out and retool. Although grad school's changeable and bendable schedules are gone, no matter your past, you likely know how to show up for a job and do your time.

But your first job in this new profession as a therapist might feel a bit different. Not only is there the understandable angst of starting out, but you also have to readjust to what writer David Foster Wallace called the "day in, day out" of your new workday world. Before, even though you may have gotten into a heated argument with your partner right before heading off to campus, had kids throwing up in the middle of the night, or had a "hard" night of going out with friends, you could likely coast through your classes, mindlessly turn over garden soil, or shuffle enough papers to get through the day sitting in your cubby at the bank.

What's different now is that coasting is not an option. You're no longer "just the student," no longer slinging cappuccinos, planting azaleas, or sifting through loan applications. Now you have to be on point. Now you have not just customers who have been waiting in line for ten minutes, but *clients* who have been waiting for three weeks, maybe longer, and who have taken personal time off from work to see you or someone like you. They have complicated stories and needs, they remind you a little too much of your parents or your ex, and truth be told, adding fuel to the fire, you really don't have any idea of how to help them.

Just as they don't care if their doctor hasn't been sleeping well, they don't care about your sick kids, rough nights, or newbie insecurity. They expect and need you to be alert, engaged, and ready to offer sage advice. By the end of that 50-minute session, they expect to feel better—less worried, more hopeful, and holding some mental health equivalent of a prescription with clear next steps.

Too Many Masters

But wait, there's more. If these demands are not enough for you to adjust to, you also have someone looking over your shoulder, someone else you need to please: your supervisor. Sure, you've had other bosses in the past, but the learning curve was probably less steep, the ultimate responsibility less heavy. And although your supervisor seems supportive, you know that she too, like all bosses, has her own pressures—she also didn't sleep well, had sick kids or grouchy partners. Still, she's showing up and stepping up, and she expects you to do the same. She needs to have your charts up-to-date because an audit is due from the state or because her boss is breathing down her neck after getting burned more than a few times; she's learned that policy is policy, and policy is important. That stack of forms that clutter her desk is, she lets you know, actually important to someone somewhere. So you need to check those boxes, get those progress notes in by Friday at 4:00 P.M., and follow up with the client's psychiatrist to make sure there's an appointment documented in his file.

New Kid on the Block

You sit in group supervision or a staff meeting, and not only do you not know everybody and feel like that new kid on the block, but you're worried about what others think of you. Even though you know you should know better, you really do feel like an eight-year-old hanging out with a group of teenagers who are all best friends. You feel a bit intimidated; you worry that you'll say something stupid, and everyone will roll their eyes and giggle under their breath.

Know What You Don't Know: Impostor Syndrome

If worrying about what your peers think isn't enough of a concern, there's always the sense that it's only a matter of time before you're going to get busted by your clients—that they're going to see through your veneer of bravado, call you on the fact that you don't know what you're doing. And most of the time, you don't. You're not sure about what you know, but clearly know what you don't know, which is a lot—like what to do with your 4:00 P.M. appointment with a child with attention-deficit disorder, or how to keep your therapy notes within the box on the electronic record software, or whether Ann, your client, was upset by your last-session parting comment. It's that same feeling you had in the tenth grade when you tried to bs your answer about what happened in Chapter Three of *The Catch in the Rye* when you hadn't even read the first page. You're disoriented, overwhelmed.

Welcome to your new world, where the expectations and stakes are suddenly higher. Time to control what you can control and for some tips to help you make this transition.

Clarify Work Expectations

Your supervisor realizes that you're starting out, that your skill level is not the same as Cloe, who's been there for ten years, and that it will take you a few months to get your sea legs. But to help rein in your runaway anxiety, get that reality check. If you are on probation and worried about what you must do to pass it, put the problem to rest. Ask your supervisor what you're being evaluated on. She'll likely pull out the evaluation form, and you'll find that the expectations have to do with coming to work on time, meeting baseline clinical skills—nothing about getting five stars on Google reviews or curing cancer. Good to know. Take a deep breath.

Establish Three- to Six-Month Goals

Because your brain is scrambling and you're feeling like you need to know and do everything, sitting down with your supervisor and coming up with reasonable goals for the next few months will help you focus on what is important rather than feeling that everything is. Having five things on your list rather than 50 will lower the bar and lower your anxiety.

Lean into Your Supervisor

This is tricky. Because you are sensitive to what you don't know and to being evaluated, you naturally feel you need to hold back and not ask too many clinical questions for fear of exposing your ignorance. The counterintuitive stance is to lean into your supervisor. No, you don't want to appear constantly overwhelmed, don't want to seem to be high maintenance, but you do want to ask for the help you need. Supervisors appreciate this. Why? Because part of their job is not only supporting you but maintaining quality control. And you make their job easier if you help them identify where you need to boost your competence and skill set.

Therapy is an individual sport. Just as you can wake up in the middle of the night worrying about how your client Tom is doing, your supervisor can have the same fears about what you are doing. So she wants to know as much as possible about what is going on or what you are struggling with. Just as you don't want to have any surprises about the state of Tom, she doesn't want to have any surprises about you and what you are doing with Tom. Supervisors appreciate your openness; it helps them with their anxiety. This is about building trust all around.

Ask for a Three-Month Informal Evaluation

A good supervisor will be giving you feedback regularly. But to help you not worry about any surprises springing up, ask if you can have an informal evaluation at the halfway point in your probationary period so you can be reassured and fine-tune what you have been doing.

Know Your Supervisor's Availability and Expectations

If you worry that you may be bothering your supervisor too much or seem too needy, ask your supervisor about her availability: yes, it is okay to come in to see me if my door is open, or no, write down your questions and we will talk about them when we meet on Thursday at 9:00. Also find out about her supervisory style: come in with an agenda, start by giving me a rundown on the status of your cases, or no, she is more laid-back, and supervisory sessions can be more free flowing. Don't guess; find out.

Ask for the Specific Help You Need

Even if your supervisor seems laid-back, her time is still limited. To maximize your time, do come to supervision with specific questions. Yes, sometimes you need to vent; sometimes you may want to walk through a difficult session in detail. But if you need detailed first aid information, ask for it. Tell her you need guidelines on assessing your new client's anxiety or suggestions about what to ask to confirm that a six-year-old may have an attention problem. Yes, you're showing your vulnerabilities, but you are also proactive and honest. Your supervisor will appreciate that.

Help Your Supervisor Understand How You Learn Best

Most folks have their own learning style. Some learn by reading books, some by watching videos, others by observing colleagues, and still others by doing role plays. Some therapists like to map out a possible treatment plan in advance with a supervisor, whereas others like to wing it and use supervision to mop up after. Let your supervisor know what works for you.

Get to Know Your Colleagues

And because doing therapy is a solo act, it helps to feel that you are part of a team. Your colleagues may not have your back the way your supervisor does, but, like siblings, they can help you weather the day-to-day. Again, you may be reluctant to open up for fear of their judgment or you may be shy, but you can set the pace. Now is the time to begin to replace the buddies you may have lost.

You're going through a big transition. The key to managing your anxiety is being proactive, saying and getting what you need, and realizing that others' expectations are likely not as demanding as your own.

What do you need most to feel settled in this new profession?

CHAPTER 5

Piling On

Common Clinical Challenges

If making the transition to your job isn't already enough of a challenge, we've got a few more challenges to add to your pile, those connected to your clinical work itself. Here are some of the common ones that you're likely to face.

You Feel Overwhelmed by Content

In my clinical supervision training, I ask the audience of supervisors: And what do the progress notes of new clinicians look like? Invariably, someone immediately yells out, "Long!" And they typically are long, for several reasons. One is that clients come to sessions loaded down with stories—blow-by-blow accounts of who said what and when, mountains of background information, or a seemingly endless list of problems that need to be addressed now; it hits you like a tidal wave. In your efforts to be a good listener, you tend to be reactive than proactive; rather than shaping the conversation, you take what you get. And even if you wanted to be more assertive, you might still have trouble. It's likely you lack the filters you need to sort what is important information and what is not. Your anxiety, like your clients', makes everything feel important. No wonder you spend the session essentially taking dictation, writing down everything the client says, and then copying it all into your notes.

The end result is that you wind up with two tons of content dropped in your lap and feeling like your clients—overwhelmed with not one problem but several and flooded by contradictory stories that they and now you are struggling to sort out.

You Wrestle with Time Management

With so much content coming at you, reining it all in becomes a problem. When I started working, I would run over most of my sessions, and by the afternoon, the minutes stacked up; I was a half-hour or more behind schedule. Partly this was due to my not wanting to cut clients off; I had a hard time saying that our time was up. But it was also my problem with judging time. I'd make the mistake of asking Ms. Jones five minutes before the end of the hour about the results of her mother's blood test or inquire about "the tragedy" that she had just mentioned. She would now emotionally fall apart, and I would spend fifteen minutes helping her calm down. I hadn't developed the skill of pacing.

You Can Diagnose but Get Stumped on Treatment

Sam is clearly depressed—lying in bed for long hours, a why-bother attitude toward everything, and filled with regrets about his past. Molly says she is fed up with her relationship and wants out—she's tired of her boyfriend always getting stoned and playing video games like she's not even there. Six-year-old Allie is struggling at school. Her teachers think she may be hyperactive, aka attention-deficit/hyperactivity disorder (ADHD), and her parents agree that she never sits still and can't focus on her homework. Jake says he's been waking up at 3:00 A.M. every day worrying about everything under the sun; he's been doing it forever, but it's gotten worse.

Okay, you agree that Sam is depressed. Molly needs some support and advice on navigating her relationship, Allie probably does have ADHD, and Jake may have some generalized anxiety disorder. Good job. But now the hard part: What do you do when you meet with them next week to begin to fix these problems? This is where the going can get tough.

You're Facing New Clinical Problems

Intake has passed along to you some new cases: A teen who has been losing weight because she has been restricting; an adult male who thinks he has a porn addiction; parents who are concerned that their son is encopretic and other kids are making fun of him. You shake your head and feel overwhelmed. This is stuff you don't remember ever learning about in grad school or your fieldwork. Yes, you read a chapter in a textbook about eating disorders; you have a vague memory of a video about addictions. But they're showing up this week, and the teenager is already here. Panic is understandable.

There's Too Much Emotion

You are seeing Jim and Melissa for the first time in couple therapy. It's clear that Jim really doesn't want to be there—he avoids eye contact, jiggles his leg, and interrupts Melissa every third sentence. And then she brings up last Christmas, and he hits the roof—"There you go again! I'm tired of this sh**." And Jim stomps out, slamming the door behind him. Or, it's not about Jim and Melissa, but a teen who is determined to cry forever over a breakup despite what you say or do, or a grandfather who goes on a five-minute rant in a remote family session, then says his chest hurts, and suddenly evaporates from the computer screen. You're overwhelmed; you're shell-shocked.

You're Being Overresponsible

If you feel your skills are shaky, are feeling performance pressure, yet are filled with passion and idealism and are sensitive and empathic, it's easy to do too much. I've supervised new clinicians who lent clients money, transported the family's dog to the vet, and found a used couch to replace the client's broken-down one, trying to borrow an agency truck to deliver it to them on the weekend. If all or any of these demands are part of your job description, go for it. But most often, these were acts of kindness driven by compassion and anxiety and well outside the therapist's job description.

Maybe your personality gives you a stronger-than-usual tendency to take responsibility. If you are an only child or a first-born child, or if there was at least a six-year gap between you and your older sibling, if you were the kid who always did well in school and felt the pressure of needing to do well, if you're self-critical, tend to avoid confrontation, have a lot of "shoulds" in your head, welcome to the world of therapists. All too many of us grew up in families where there was chaos created by an addicted or emotionally unstable parent, impossibly high expectations, or ever-present tension that left us constantly walking on eggshells and adapting an "I'm happy if you're happy" stance. Being the good kids that so many of us were meant to be, we learned early on to be sensitive to the needs and demands of others. While being sensitive is good for creating the foundation of empathy so crucial in our work, it also fuels that low tolerance for strong emotions. "Making you happy" means avoiding confrontation and always accommodating.

And if you're accommodating, you're not setting boundaries. Rather than actively shaping the session, it's easy to lapse into passivity. If you're worried about making clients happy, you tend to be overresponsible. You work harder than they do; you worry about them more than they are worried about themselves. And if you have an intimidating supervisor, it's the worst of all possible worlds. You believe your supervisor will be happy with you if your clients are happy with you. You're caught in a vise where pleasing everyone around you becomes your primary goal. Rather than focusing on your clients and helping them realize where they are getting stuck in running their own lives, you're instead focusing on saving yourself from your own anxiety.

This all makes sense but can get in the way of doing good therapy. The purpose of therapy isn't about pleasing.

If any of this resonates, don't despair. Your reactions may make your work more difficult than it needs to be; you may feel like you are carrying too much on your shoulders all the time (and you are); you may not be as effective or efficient as you'd like to be. This is what makes starting out difficult. But know that you're not a lousy therapist. You're just a new therapist, and as you gain experience and mature professionally and personally, much of this tendency to do too much will recede. It's simply a matter of time. You likely have plenty of time to grow . . . and you will.

But until you get there, you can still do a lot right now to reduce your anxiety and move the process along.

Build Your Skills

Here you want to do what we discussed in the last chapter—have honest conversations with your supervisor about your clinical needs, and set those three- to six-month goals. Your supervisor can help you set priorities for training based on your skill level and agency needs. Develop treatment maps for specific diagnoses, so you're not fumbling through the treatment phase with clients. With your supervisor's help, have clear goals for each session so you're not doing cookie-cutter therapy, going on autopilot, falling into an accommodating, little-kid role, or seeming passive.

Realize That Others Don't See You the Way You See Yourself

I have a tree-size plant that sits right behind me in my office. After a few sessions or even months, I've had clients ask whether that plant is new. Obviously, it's not new, but I always take it as a sign that they are getting better—they are less focused on themselves and are beginning to look around and notice the bigger world.

You are not as transparent as you feel: No one sees your fluttering heart nor hears your stumbling words. This is true with colleagues and especially true with clients. They are usually so naturally focused on their own anxiety and how they present themselves that they barely notice you.

Work Up Lines about Your Experience

You want to help clients feel safe partly by letting them know you are competent. Here it's helpful, so you're not thinking on your feet and fumbling about, to come up with a solid description of your experience and approach—research you've done, experience with clients, and situations like theirs. Plan out what you'll say so you remember to include things you might forget in the heat of the moment. Doing so helps you feel more empowered and in control and counter concerns clients may think about but won't say.

Dress Up

Power suits and personal armor are okay. You cannot not make a first impression; these nonverbal messages to the clients carry some weight.

Be Proactive in Sessions

This is about sculpting the process. Yes, you want to be an empathic yet active listener. But laying back and asking how you feel, being reactive through those initial sessions, is not only what clients aren't wanting but conveys a passivity and perhaps insecurity. Go proactive. Don't overcontrol the session but do step up and shape it. It lets clients know that despite what you worry they are thinking—that you are too young or inexperienced—you are in charge and know what you're doing.

Leadership helps clients feel safe. This is particularly important when sitting across from clients who remind you of your parents.

Craft Educational Speeches

No, you don't need to do a 30-minute speech about the impact of anxiety on the brain. Still, even ten-minute speeches about their presenting concerns—their child with ADHD, their brain on anxiety or withdrawal from alcohol, the common emotional wounds or dysfunctional communication patterns couples can fall into—are almost always appreciated. Not only do you place their problems into the range of the common and ordinary, but you are helping them make sense of their experience in a new way. And, as a by-product, you're not only scrambling to think on your feet, but you feel empowered by simply letting them know important information they probably don't know. They walk out seeing you as someone who knows his stuff.

Change Your Story

You think you had a productive session with your client last week, but now he suddenly cancels or doesn't show up. Your head may become self-critical, obsessing, replaying what you might have done wrong that you didn't realize.

Stop. Don't go down that rabbit hole. Yes, it may be about you, but the reality check is that it probably is not; unfortunately, you and therapy are often not as important to clients as they are to you. They get derailed by running late at work and having sick kids, or their ADHD causes them to be disorganized and forgetful; their elderly parent has fallen and broken her hip, and therapy has slipped to the bottom of their to-do list. Call them and check it out. Try believing what they say rather than lapsing into your story about yourself.

Work on You

If you feel your "I'm happy if you're happy" stance is interfering with your work too much—if you are feeling burned out or carrying your job in your head home with you every day, or if your intolerance for strong emotions keeps you on edge or passive—you may want to consider supplementing your skill building with some personal therapy.

This will speed up your growth and provide support and the tools to help lower your anxiety.

See what works for you. It's about skills and anxiety—yours and theirs—and the theme here is that you want to learn to manage yours by approaching it and then deliberately shaping it. With a bit of faking-it-till-you-make-it, you will eventually make it.

You are already a sensitive and empathic healer. What do you need to feel more empowered?

CHAPTER 6

Reflections

My First Year

I'm sitting in the middle of the family's living room, in a house at the end of a dirt road somewhere in South Carolina. The father is sitting on the couch, leaning forward, arms resting on his knees, his shirt unbuttoned for some reason, revealing a long scar down the center of his chest. His wife sits next to him, wringing her hands in slow motion. Their eight-year-old son is darting around the edges of the room. (Why isn't he in school?) I'm sitting in the chair opposite them, my clipboard at the ready, and, of course, wearing a suit—maybe a bit overdressed, especially since there is no air conditioning. To add to the ambience, *The 700 Club*, a daily Christian TV talk show, is not quite blaring in the background but close. I'm here because the family doesn't have a car, and the guidance counselor at the boy's school made a referral to our agency.

"The problem with Billy," says Dad, "is that this boy was allergic to soy milk. You see, when he was a baby, he couldn't drink regular milk, and the doctor said we needed to switch to soy milk. It's the soy milk that messed up his head." The mother glances at her husband, then me, then nods.

He's answering my question about why he thinks his son has been acting up in class and getting numerous referrals to the principal's office. It sounds like the dad is bypassing any psychosocial explanation I might have going through my head and sees the boy's behavioral problems as caused by soy-milk-induced brain damage. Not only does this problem sound serious to the dad, but it also sounds pretty unrepairable—a done deal. "Actually," he says, "I've already said this to the school folks. I don't know why you're out here." I'm now starting to ask myself the same question, feeling both stumped and stupid.

Looking back on it, I realize now that the father was actually partially correct—maybe it wasn't the soy milk that "messed up" his son's brain, but he likely had a "brain" problem, namely, ADHD. But back then, there was no such thing as ADHD. Instead, there was "minimal brain damage," a scary-sounding condition of unknown origin that mysteriously caused some children to perseverate and be unusually active. The good news at the time was that somebody thought the children would somehow outgrow this condition when they hit puberty (they didn't). And, by the way, there was also no borderline personality, no posttraumatic stress, no self-harm, and nothing anyone would be willing to call child abuse. The DSM world was short and simple—there were a few types of psychoses and neuroses, and the real cause of schizophrenia was those "schizophrenogenic" mothers who "messed up" their kids' heads by being alternatingly distant and intrusive, critical and positive. Prozac and its kin were still in the fruit-fly testing stage, and the range of psychotropic medications was limited: there was Thorazine . . . and Thorazine. Oh, wait, we also had "electric shock." It was the Dark Ages.

Of course, we didn't think that way at the time. We, in the therapy world, were the enlightened ones, on the cutting edge of the cutting edge. Freud and psychoanalysis were being pushed to the side by behaviorism and family therapy. Experiential therapies, such as Gestalt, where clients talked to empty chairs or reenacted their dreams in a session, were hot, along with lots of guided imagery, and even having clients sit on your lap as part of a "reparenting" process.

But I can't use the times to excuse my novice (and normal) ineptness. Not that I wasn't trying—did I say I had a suit and a clipboard? But that first year for me was a series of blurs. Talking to parents who looked like my parents and hearing their opening question: "You got kids?" Fortunately, my 25-year-old self could truthfully squeak out that I did. But that didn't get me off the hook: "But you're only, what, eighteen? What the hell do you know about raising kids?!"

Back in my office, I can't say I felt much more on top of things professionally. At the end of a session with an attractive woman around my age who was getting divorced, she casually asked if we could maybe go out for coffee sometime after one of our sessions. Or, after realizing in my first session with 45-year-old Ed that the poor guy was horribly depressed (go me!), I started the second session by asking, "So how have you been feeling this past week?" "Depressed." I realized that Ed and I had pretty much reached the end of any productive conversation; I just maxed out my intervention skills. Once again, I felt stumped and stupid.

I did have supervisory support, and as luck would have it, my supervisor was not only a pioneer in bringing therapy into people's homes, and in raising the community's awareness of child abuse and racial inequality, but she was also a generous, warm-hearted, old-school social worker who did a wonderful job at helping me feel safe and supported. Despite that, I felt intimidated. In my mind, I was hanging on by a thread, and it was only a matter of time before she would realize that I didn't know what I was doing and I would get busted and summarily marched out of the building. The less I said, I figured, the better. I might be able to eke out a bit more time to get those job applications to Home Depot and Piggly Wiggly.

So, while I said as little as possible to my supervisor, I did say more to my colleagues. Unfortunately, a couple of them were just like me, new graduates; the best we could do for each other was mumble in the hallways about how we had no idea what we were going to do with the new couple coming in five minutes, like high schoolers sweating over next period's algebra exam. But there was an older woman, the grandmother at the agency, who I did get up the courage to ask in whispered tones about Ed: "So, I'm seeing this guy who I know is depressed, but . . . what do I actually do in the session?"

But as the year unfolded, the sessions seemed to get a bit easier—I started getting my sea legs and, most surprisingly, despite me, so did some of my clients. I suggested that the grumbling parents use a reward chart (that I had read about the night before) with their "lazy" daughter who wasn't doing her chores. Not only did the parents try it, but they said it worked. Though I turned down the coffee date with the woman who was getting divorced, she stuck around and, after a few sessions of chatter about her SOB husband, unexpectedly and tearfully disclosed that she had been sexually abused as a child, a secret she had never shared with anyone until that very moment. I realized that maybe my clients weren't seeing me as I saw myself. I certainly didn't have all the answers, but perhaps I wasn't quite as stupid as I felt.

PART II

YOUR WORK

There's plenty of information about how to be a therapist. The challenge is learning to be the therapist you want to be—the one that builds on your personality, strengths, passions, and visions. That is a goal you will hopefully discover and reach as you move forward and experiment in your work. This part offers tidbits of clinical ideas to help you along the way. Some you may discard, and others keep—that's fine. Discovery really is about experimenting.

CHAPTER 7

Six Ways to Build Rapport

You know about building rapport, especially when starting with a new client. Here at their first session, you ask Dan what he does for work; Ann about her life as an artist and how she learned to create art; their daughter, what school she goes to, her best friend's name, and whether she has any pets. You're chatting, helping the client or clients settle in and feel comfortable. You're done.

Maybe, maybe not. Chatting may be the first step in connecting, but ultimately rapport is about laying down the foundation of what is to become the therapeutic relationship; rapport is about safety. Clients need to feel that they are in good hands, that you're competent, that they like you, and feel they can trust you. So, if you want to take rapport to the next level, here are a few suggestions to add to your skill-and-style toolbox.

1. Actively Listen

Active listening is more than sitting up straight, stone-faced with occasional nods of your head. And it is more than saying, "I understand," which can often sound formulaic. Instead, active listening is about being . . . active, fully engaging with clients to gather the information you need. It might sound like this: "I understand what you said, but I'm not sure what you meant. Can you tell me more . . . ?" You acknowledge the emotions underlying their statements: "Cindy, it must be frustrating for you"; "Luis, you sound really worried about your son."

Actively listening is probably the most basic and powerful means of building rapport. Many clients feel constantly dismissed in their closest relationships; in therapy, they finally feel that they are heard, that what they say matters. The good family physician does this when she asks what's wrong and takes the time to sincerely listen to what you have to say.

2. Show Leadership

If active listening is atop the list of rapport-building techniques, leadership is second. It's less specific, broader. You show competence by acting competent, which usually translates into stepping up and stepping forward. Clients are coming to you not to chat but for guidance based on your expertise. They need to hear what you think, but are also wondering in those initial sessions whether you have the will and power to deliver what they expect. Leadership is not about micromanaging the process or going on and on about your expertise and skill, but about shaping what unfolds rather than being passive; about providing feedback in those first sessions so clients know you understand their problems and can offer something—clear directives, new ways of seeing the problem, options for solving their problems in better ways. Don't just nod your head and then thank them for coming.

3. Highlight Similarities

People feel more comfortable with people who are like them, and some clients can be aggressive in finding this out: "So, do you have kids?" But rather than going reactive, go proactive. Luis says that he was in the military, and you mention in a sentence or two that you were in the military too, or that you grew up in a military family. Tan says he went to school in Michigan, and you tell him your father grew up in Michigan. Or your last names are ethnically similar, and you ask where his family of origin is from. Or Cindy says her five-month-old is still waking up many times during the night and wearing her out, and you briefly relate how your second child did the same, and that you remember difficult it was.

This is not about making the conversation about you or fictionalizing your background but intentionally looking for overlap and possible shared experiences. By highlighting these similarities, you increase that human-to-human connection; you become less a stranger.

4. Be Sensitive to Differences

Our society has become increasingly sensitive to differences in so many areas—culture, gender, race, religion—and so has clinical practice. Familiarizing yourself with these differences is an important foundation for your work. That said, you don't need an encyclopedic knowledge of various cultural values, but rather a respectful attitude. This means noticing and commenting, showing curiosity and interest in differences rather than dismissing them. You can demonstrate this simply by asking questions: "You mentioned that you are Hindu [or Muslim or Jewish or born-again Christian]. Can you tell me how your religious beliefs shape your values?"; "What pronouns would you like me to use?"; "Because I am not Chinese myself, I wonder if you can tell me how your heritage and upbringing have influenced you the most." Clients appreciate the opportunity to discuss their particular views of life. By asking and listening carefully, you show that you respect their opinions and unique perspectives and are willing to incorporate them into your working partnership.

5. Match Body Posture, Voice Tone, Language, and Perceptual Systems

If you mirror the body posture of your client, crossing your legs, leaning forward like she is doing while talking, she will feel more connected. Ditto, if you match the client's tone: the energy of the six-year-old, the quiet hunched-over sound of the teen. If your client throws in cuss words, throw in a couple yourself, or if a scientist starts talking about research findings, do the same. Use the skills of neurolinguistic programming and speak the language of each person's perceptual system: "Tan, how do you *see* the problem?"; "Cindy, how do you *feel* when the baby won't settle"; "Luis, how do you *handle* it when your son blows up at you?" Connecting this way is another form of building on similarities.

6. Listen for Transference Cues

You are undoubtedly familiar with the concept of transference—that clients always look at you through the lens of their past and present relationships. If a client had a critical dad, he is understandably sensitive to criticism from others; or if she felt neglected by her mother because the mother was an alcoholic, those childhood wounds can carry over to the present where a text that goes unanswered for 20 minutes feels like rejection or triggers panic.

Knowing that transference is part of the therapeutic process can help you be sensitive to possible reactions down the road. But you can also usually and quickly uncover cues—transference cues—even in the first session. When Nan says that her mom has been so supportive because she checks on her every day; that her father was always so impatient and wouldn't let her finish a sentence before he interrupted her; that her ex-husband was so passive and just sat there—you now have quickly learned how to be and not be. Be more like mom, less like dad or the ex; check in, be patient, be active.

Again, rapport is about creating safety and, by being alert to potential emotional triggers, you avoid resistance and create a safe or safer relationship.

These are techniques to consider, to experiment with. Take them one at a time. See what works, what resonates with your style. The goal is to engage clients so they feel connected and safe.

CHAPTER 8

Be the Adult

One of the key advantages you have in helping your clients is that they are clients. Usually, other people in their lives step in and offer advice—sisters, parents, friends—but these other helpers are handicapped because they have a history, assumptions, and expectations; because they care so much, their anxiety understandably bleeds into their helping. You too can find yourself doing much the same if you are not careful—your own feelings and assumptions can interfere with your ability to listen and provide interventions. But by and large, you have the advantage of seeing clients more neutrally than their friends and family do. Because you have some distance and share no history, because you are outside the system, you are able to see the blind spots that they and their helpers cannot, the larger patterns and themes that get washed away in the flood of details that form their often chaotic daily lives. This vantage point, along with your copy of the DSM and your clinical approach, create your "clinical" perspective, your unbiased view that gives them a new lens through which to view their concerns.

As we discussed earlier, when you're starting out, despite having these tools, the assessment process can feel overwhelming—facts and stories to sort through, history to consider—and it's easy to feel like your clients: flooded with problems, situations, and emotions. Here is a simple, commonsense lens to help you quickly define clients and their issues and map out a preliminary treatment plan. Try it out, see if it is helpful and if it can be another tool to add to your clinical toolbox.

Be Adult

While I don't follow Murray Bowen's (1993) overall approach to family therapy, two of his concepts are ones that I've used over the years. One is his notion of having the client become the change agent for the family or system: If one person can step up and change the dysfunctional patterns of the system, and hold steady despite expected opposition, the other members of the system have to change in some way. This is empowering, especially when you see an individual who feels helpless to change the dynamics of relationships, be it a couple, family, or larger system like a workplace.

His other concept that has always resonated with me is that of the differentiated self, what I've come to call over the years "the adult." This is one that I always lean upon. Here Bowen offers a model of how to be in relationships, one that is unentangled, that unlocks "enmeshment" with its blurry boundaries and codependency and that sidesteps the common emotional potholes that Bowen saw as handicapping individual and family success. Here are its basic components (Gilbert, 1992; Taibbi, 2019):

- An ability to be emotionally calm
- An ability to observe yourself in a relationship pattern and make changes without expectations of the other
- An ability to view others as anxious or fearful rather than as malicious or manipulative
- An ability to not react in kind to the anger or anxiety of others
- An ability to make choices and be assertive even if this risks the approval or acceptance of others
- An ability to focus more on your personal responsibility and behavior than on the behavior of the other
- An ability to be thoughtful in decision making, to be able to solve problems as they arise

Attorneys talk about the "reasonable man" standard, in which a defendant's behavior is compared against what most of us would expect a reasonable person to do in a similar situation. What I like about the Bowen adult model is that it has that same commonsense feel; it makes sense to me on a gut level about what good mental health is about: a great mix of values and emotion regulation, courageous action, and boundary setting, along with the ability to be compassionate and generous. His model provides you with a standard against which to measure the client's emotional health quickly.

This approach, of course, is what your physician takes all the time. You come in with symptoms of exhaustion. She draws a blood sample, and off to the lab it goes. By comparing your results against a medical norm—that your red cell count is off, your vitamin D levels are down—she can narrow her focus or even diagnose the cause, all in fifteen minutes. You can do the same by comparing your client against Bowen's "adult."

Tom, for example, says he has ongoing explosive arguments with his boyfriend. Laying his story side-by-side with Bowen's adult model, the gap between them is easy to see. Unlike the adult, Tom isn't able to remain calm or resist reacting in kind to his boyfriend's upset. Or Caleb admits that he just bought a car that he really can't afford, and a bell goes off in your head that this guy is making impulsive rather than thoughtful decisions. Or, as Alicia complains yet again about her supervisor's micromanagement of her work but takes no steps toward fixing the problem, you ask yourself, "Why can't Alicia step up and be assertive?"

Again, like your physician and her lab results, you now can quickly zero in: sidestep the he-said-he-said of Tom's arguments but instead talk about his struggle with emotional regulation; avoid getting into the weeds with Caleb about why he bought that car but focus on his impulsive, emotionally driven decision making; bypass Alicia's blow-by-blow of her boss's injustice-of-the-week and ask about her seeming inability to put her problem to rest.

You have both a ready assessment tool and a preliminary treatment plan. What's not to like?

If you want to experiment with this approach, start by simply thinking in this comparative, commonsense way. As a client is describing his problems and relationships, ask yourself what is the gap, the difference between what the client is saying and doing, and what we might expect from a "reasonable" someone else? Once you've identified this difference, you can drill down to discover how and why the client thinks and acts differently.

CHAPTER 9

What Can't You Do?

In addition to Bowen's "adult" model, here's another quick assessment tool to experiment with. Stepping back, you and I can probably agree that it's likely that Tom's, Caleb's, and Alicia's presenting problems discussed in the last chapter are not isolated, situational events. Tom's problem with emotional regulation isn't limited to his boyfriend, nor is Caleb's impulsivity limited to cars, or Alicia's upset and inability to act unique to her supervisor. Their presenting problems are rooted in emotional triggers, learned coping styles, and the notion that our ways of approaching life and stress and everyday problems are not only pretty much set but spread out across the canvas of our lives.

A Buddhist saying captures these ideas in a simple sentence: How you do anything is how you do everything. This has become one of my mantras over the years, and I find myself saying it often to clients. But if you break it down, the sentence is more complex than it initially appears.

It starts with *how* you do rather than *what* you do. This is an important distinction. *How* is about process: how we cope and respond, the actions and reactions we take. Process is what we focus on in therapy and what we do in therapy—shaping the unfolding process to create an experience, whether through insight into the past, through an awareness of thoughts and feelings in the present, or through building on strengths and skills that the client is unable to see.

But many clients, particularly those new to therapy, don't think about *how* but about *what*: content. Tom talks about his boyfriend and the facts filling the argument; Caleb focuses on his car or money; Alicia thinks about the supervisor, the micromanagement. They want to fix the *what*—the boyfriend, the facts, the money, the supervisor. But if you believe that the source of problems isn't the *what* but the *how*, that the faulty process is the source of problems and the client's struggles, you can avoid both that common start-up tendency to get sucked into and lost in the weeds of the clients' content. And you can avoid replicating the problem in the room, where you, like them, wind up feeling overwhelmed, angry, and fixated on the content. Instead, by helping clients see that the content (the facts and situations) isn't the problem but rather how they react to the problem, you and they are dealing with the source rather than with the symptoms.

But the second half of our Buddhist sentence, how you do *anything* is how you do *everything*, is equally important. We're back to the notion that coping styles reach out across the broad landscape of our lives. When you step back and survey this landscape of your past, your relationships, and the situations you decide to label as problems, where do you get stuck running your life? What can't you do? These are your meta-problems, your Achilles' heel, and just like Bowen's adult, most folks don't have dozens of them, but rather their current problems and most of those in the future can generally be reduced to a couple.

The next sections are the meta-problems that, from my experience, you are most likely to see.

Can't Tolerate Conflict and the Strong Emotions of Others

Although Alicia lays her problem in her supervisor's lap, we wouldn't be surprised if she said she had had similar issues with other people in her life. Her meta-problem—her what-can't-she-do, her stuckpoint—is that she can't tolerate the conflict or the potential strong negative emotions of others. Alicia sweeps problems under the rug, or blames herself, to avoid confrontation. She accommodates, internalizes, and walks on eggshells. Because she can't move toward her anxiety, she can only freeze or flee.

For clients dealing with this faulty process, the consequences are many and significant. Unsolved problems accumulate and, as they do, clients become increasingly overwhelmed. This, in turn, often creates a long laundry list of problems, particularly for those clients in crisis, that they hand to you in their first session. Or they are overwhelmed by trying to juggle the varying demands of all the masters they are trying to please. Or depression sets in because they either feel trapped in their lives or are essentially living the lives of others rather than their own. And finally, this suppression can back up on them: Alicia cuts, periodically goes on a drinking binge, or reaches some breaking point where she simply walks off her job.

By recognizing that avoiding conflict is Alicia's Achilles' heel, you now have a treatment goal, namely, to help her stop doing all of the above: stop walking on eggshells, stop biting her tongue, stop accommodating and going along with, stop avoiding and shutting down. Instead, Alicia needs to do what she can't do: speak up, tell others what she needs and, most of all, learn to tolerate strong emotions and conflict by moving through them (and finding out that she survived). By having such corrective emotional experiences, she begins to heal her past and reduce those childhood-based fears. It's as simple and as hard as that. If you can help Alicia change this meta-problem, she is essentially done with therapy. Like the rest of us, she will undoubtedly continue to have situational challenges in her life; by fixing this primary meta-problem, the knot that keeps her from dealing with those challenges effectively will be untied. Alicia will handle problems in a new way, which will ripple across the other areas of her life. She will run her life better.

The beauty of this treatment path is that because it is not situational but all-encompassing, Alicia can start anywhere. The target problem is not about the current situation but about her. If she's not ready to go head-to-head with her supervisor, she can take a baby step of saying no to volunteering on that committee at work or of confronting her partner about getting his stuff off the dining room table. And it's okay if it takes her a few days to figure out how she feels or get up the courage to act; she can even send an email or text if face-to-face still feels too intimidating. It doesn't matter *what* Alicia does as long as she focuses on the *how* and does what's difficult for her to do.

Can't Regulate Emotions

Tom can't control his anger; Caleb's emotionally driven and impulsive. As with Alicia, your treatment path is clear—shift from the what to the how. Move away from Tom's blaming of his boyfriend and Caleb's money issues and redefine the problem: help both be less emotionally driven; help Tom to learn to regulate his emotions, Caleb his impulsivity. Get buy-in on your assessment, and then focus on the process: Explore with Tom the triggers for his anger and with Caleb what sparks his impulsiveness. See if they can tell when their rational brains are going off-line and their emotions are driving the train. Explore the source in the past, or teach skills to lower the emotional temperature. Solve these bigger problems so they can solve the smaller, presenting ones.

Can't Tolerate Making Mistakes

Michelle says she has trouble making decisions. You may begin to think she is struggling like Alicia—that when decisions involve other people, she becomes afraid of upsetting them and so waffles or caves in. But as you dig deeper, you find it's not others she is trying to keep at bay but that always-running critical voice in her head. She just can't march ahead and make a decision; she can only move forward when she knows her decision is "right"—no mistakes allowed.

This is where Michelle, and others like her, winds up spending hours trolling through the internet to find the best dog food on the planet, where perfectionism has her double- and triple-check her emails, the spreadsheets at work, the sweater she's trying to match with a skirt. Michelle's "what can't she do" is to tolerate not being right and perfect. Her challenge is to lower her expectations, take the risk of being more spontaneous, and realize that all decisions don't carry the same weight and that almost all mistakes can be repaired. If she can continue becoming less perfectionistic with your support, that critical voice will eventually subside.

Your support may be challenging Michelle to push against her anxiety and pick one dog food on the first page of Google. You help her see that this is a first-world problem rather than the end-of-the-world decision it feels like to her. You introduce a dose of reality by letting her know that she can send the dog food back or buy a different one if it doesn't work, and that's okay. You also give Michelle homework about practicing making decisions quickly and being more spontaneous by trusting her gut. You show her ways of pushing back against the critical voice or exploring its source in her past.

Can't Let Go of the Past

Adim's words are always in the past tense. He talks over and over about what he didn't do, what he should have said. His past fills his mind and life. Those who focus on the past—grudges or regrets—lose sight of the present and future and are often depressed. Like Michelle, they may also be self-critical; like Alicia, they may suppress their needs and emotions. Or the underlying issue may be about trauma—flashbacks from childhood or war zones or getting suddenly fired after a 20-year career. Or about grief, what never was said and resolved.

As with many clients, Adim's stuckpoint is the belief that the only way out is to somehow reshuffle past events. But the past is closed, and the shuffling can go on forever. In other cases, clients focused on the past realize they can't go back and conclude they are doomed to feeling hopeless and depressed.

Here again, the way out that you can offer is to help them focus on this larger, underlying process. No, you can't change your past, but you can change your perception of the past in the present and the importance you are placing on it. Some clients can do this through emotional closure—reaching out, saying what they never had the chance to, or stepping up and gathering the courage to talk about their regrets or guilt. If the objects of their regret are no longer reachable, your clients can get out of their heads and get things off their chest through letter writing or expressing those deeper emotions in therapy. In this way they can begin to realize that they did the best they could, and that it's time to forgive and accept forgiveness.

Or maybe it's not about a lack of closure, but instead a sense that there is a lack of a present or future. If the present is filled with problems or emptiness, the future with fear and dread, there is nowhere else to go but into the past. And so, you try to pull yourself and the client out of the weeds of the content of the past. You help the client take action to get closure, to change his story, but also help him move forward by clearing away the obstacles cluttering the present, by becoming more mindful. You challenge the client to envision a future free of the weight of the past challenge of depressive, trapped, self-critical thinking.

Again, regardless of a client's particular answers to the question—what can't you do?—the answer and antidote, irrespective of your clinical approach, are what is at the heart of doing therapy: Whatever the route, it ultimately is about helping the client do different rather than do right; do what you avoid doing; actively push against old assumptions and behaviors. If you learn to do what you currently can't do, you change the core of yourself, your "How you do anything is how you do everything." You repair your faulty process, how you run *your* life—not someone else's life, not your past life—and run it more effectively. You become who you are.

What's your Achilles' heel, your meta-problem? What can't you do?

CHAPTER 10

Coping with Anxiety

Approach, Avoid, or Bind?

Face it, life in the therapy world is filled with anxiety—sometimes yours, and always the clients' or families'. While there's plenty of information available on various types of anxiety, and how to diagnose and treat them, early in my career I stumbled on a simple model, another quick tool. Two clinicians, Mueller and Kell (1972), developed this model. Basically, they said there are three ways to cope with anxiety: approach, avoid, and bind. Here are the characteristics of each one.

Approach

Approachers are folks who feel anxious, but they've also learned early on that anxiety is part of either learning a new skill or solving a problem. This learning likely came from parents who modeled this behavior but were patient with their child—helped her remain calm and move forward when learning, say, the nightmare of fractions. As a result, the child learned to trust and ask for help; the child learned resiliency. With this foundation in place, when anxiety arises—feeling overwhelmed tackling that new software on the job or dealing with a client who shoots down any suggestion you make—you take a few deep breaths and say to yourself, "This new software right now feels overwhelming, but I know that I'm not alone, other colleagues are undoubtedly feeling the same way, and probably in a couple of weeks I'll get this down, and I can always call up IT and get help." Or you say,

"I'm getting resistance from my client; I'm not sure why, but I can talk this out with my supervisor and see if we can come up with some better ways of addressing this."

Approachers tend to be creative, and often experimenters and risk takers.

Avoid

Avoiders are likely a majority of the clients you will see for problems with anxiety or its by-products—problems on the job, in relationships, and with physical health. Where approachers have learned to see anxiety as a by-product of other problems, for avoiders, the *feeling* of anxiety is the problem: It's always right there in their face, messing up their lives. And because it is the feeling itself that is the problem rather than the situation, their reaction is that they have to kill it—take medication or drugs—or most often avoid it: Feeling anxious about going to that party where you really don't know anyone? Text and say you're sick. Afraid to follow up on that email from your boss? Don't even look at it; push it to the side.

Bind

Binders can be tricky. When I do workshops on clinical supervision, I always tell the supervisors in the audience that you have to be careful because you can be seduced by job applicants who are binders. They often sound smart, cite research and methods, and *are* smart. But they also tend to be rigid. They tend to think in black–white terms, have a particular model or way of thinking and of doing things, and apply their approach across the board to everyone who sits in their office. And if their approach doesn't fit the problem or their clients, they blame the clients and rationalize that they were resistant.

Their solution to the problem of coping with anxiety is to live within a small comfort zone, whether it be in terms of ideas or behaviors. And it works; unlike the approachers or avoiders, binders don't feel anxious. What you might notice in clients who are binders is that they appear calm and logical. If you raise a potentially anxiety-provoking topic—"So how's your sex life?"—they will usually avoid the question and shift topics or seem not to hear what you are saying. Their partners will often complain about their control and their rigidity.

Closing the Gap

As we saw in Chapter 8 ("Be the Adult") and in Chapter 9 ("What Can't You Do?"), here you have yet another quick way of assessing clients: How do they manage their anxiety? You can quickly discern their style by the problems they present and by asking a few simple questions about how they solve problems. With this information in hand, you now have an outline of a treatment goal—closing the gap between where they are and where they know to go. Where do they get stuck in running their lives? They need to change their perspective and see anxiety the way approachers do, as a natural reaction to learning something new (including the new skills you are trying to teach them) or to solving the problem.

Your mission is to help them move forward despite how they feel. They need to take baby steps and go to that party for ten minutes or write that email back to their boss, even if you need to help them craft it. This is not about the party or the boss, you say, but about not feeling so afraid in the world, and the best way to be less afraid is not to avoid but to approach. Focus on the doing, not the outcome. Your goals are to both sell them on this underlying problem and, more important and more challenging, encourage and support them to take baby steps so that they can be successful rather than overwhelmed. Your skill comes in helping them titrate the increase in anxiety.

Because they are not feeling their anxiety, most binders are not feeling the emotional pressure to solve a problem. What may bring them in is the pressure of partners or family fed up with their rigidity and control. Even then, they may not understand the problem, blame others for being too sensitive, and see what others call rigidity and control as simply the right way to run their life.

But if they have some genuine concern and awareness, your path is equally clear. They struggle to be spontaneous, to get out of their heads and into their emotions and bodies, and to understand their partners or make changes even though they at some level care about how the other person is feeling. These clients can be difficult to work with because the key is helping them recognize their coping style and how it impacts not only those they care about, but how it is limiting their own lives as well.

Your assessment is once again determining how the client handles anxiety, broadly speaking: approach, avoid, or bind. And your treatment plan is a simple but challenging one of helping the client move toward new behaviors that are intuitively resisted.

But what about you? How do you cope with anxiety? If you buy into this model, approaching is where you want to be. This is the courage you want to develop to do the therapy you want to do, be the therapist you want to be, be confident in your own style, and be creative and curious. You not only offer clients the best of who you are, but you become a role model for managing life in a better way.

Like most of us, you probably have a primary and a secondary mode—approaching 60% of the time, but on a bad day or with certain problems or clients you can avoid or bind. That's good to know. What do you need to expand that comfort zone and be the role model and the empowered person you want to be?

CHAPTER 11

The Relationship Triangle

Bowen's adult, what can't you do, and anxiety coping styles are three effective and efficient tools for assessment and preliminary treatment. And here's yet another: the relationship triangle. It is based on the Drama Triangle, also known as the Karpman Triangle, which psychiatrist Steven Karpman (1968) developed in the late 1960s. This is my interpretation and expansion of Karpman's original ideas (Taibbi, 2022).

I think of this model as my Swiss Army knife because it incorporates so many concepts that apply to many situations. I use it in teaching clinical supervision—describing how the supervisor–clinician relationship changes over time—and as a way of explaining the dynamics of depression and anxiety: that folks who are struggling with depression or anxiety have two voices, the critical voice and the should voice, that make them feel like the victim. But one of its best uses is in describing the common sources of problems and dysfunctional patterns with couples. It not only describes what is enfolding between them and where they are struggling, but offers a road map for treatment. You'll undoubtedly see an overlap with some of the ideas we've already discussed.

Intimate Relationships

One way of depicting the dynamics of dysfunctional relationship patterns is shown in the following figure:

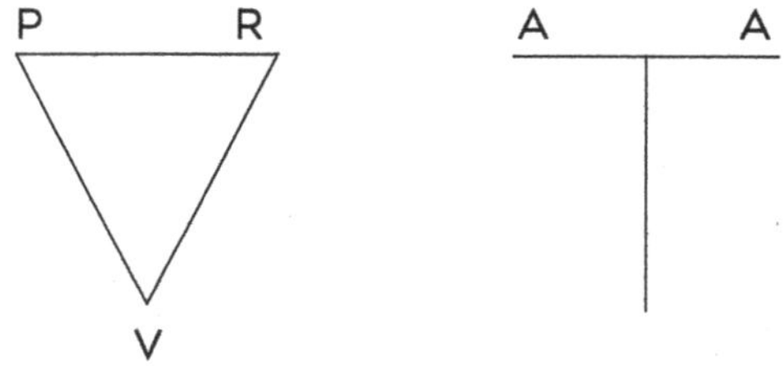

The P, R, and V represent the different roles that the people can play; here the focus is not on the people themselves, but on their roles. The roles interlock, and there is always someone on top who seems to have more power and someone on the bottom with less. The relationship moves from one vertex to the next as follows:

The person in the R position is the rescuer. The person in that role essentially has "nice guy" control. He hooks into the V, or victim. The person in that role feels overwhelmed at times. He feels that problems are falling on his head. The rescuer steps in and says, "I can help you out. Just do what I say; everything will be fine." Often couples will begin their relationship in some form of this arrangement. They psychologically cut a deal: The rescuer says I will agree to be big, strong, good, and nice; the victim says I will agree to be overwhelmed and unable to manage. Everyone is happy. The rescuer feels needed, important, and in charge. The victim has someone to take care of him.

And the arrangement works fine. Except every once in a while, one of two things happens. Sometimes the rescuer gets tired of doing it all; he feels like he is shouldering all the responsibilities and that the other is not pulling his weight, not giving anything back, not appreciating what the rescuer is doing. The rescuer gets fed up, angry, and resentful. Bam! He shifts over to the P, the persecutor role. He suddenly blows up—usually about something minor—laundry, who didn't take out the trash—or acts out—spends a lot of money, goes on a drinking binge, has an affair. He feels he deserves it; look, after all, he says to himself, at what I've been putting up with. The message underneath the behavior and anger that usually does not come out very clearly is: "Why don't you grow up! Why don't you take some responsibility! Why do I have to do everything around here! Why don't you appreciate what I am doing for you! This is unfair!" The feeling of unfairness is a strong one.

At that point, the victim gets scared and moves up to the R position, trying to make up and calm the waters. "I'm sorry," he says. "I didn't realize. I do appreciate what you do. I'll do better." Then the persecutor feels terrible about whatever he did or said and goes down to the victim's position and gets depressed. Then they both stabilize and go back to their original positions.

At other times it's the victim who gets tired of being the victim and is fed up with the other one always running the show, always telling him what to do; tired of being looked down on because the rescuer is saying, "If it weren't for me, you wouldn't make it." Bam! The victim moves to the persecutor role and, like the rescuer, blows up and gets angry or acts out, usually about something small.

The message underneath that doesn't get said is, "Why don't you get off my back! Leave me alone; stop controlling my life! Back off, I can do things myself!" The rescuer hears this and moves to the victim's position. He says to himself, "Poor me, every time I try to help, look what I get." The persecutor then feels bad about whatever he did or said and goes to the rescuer's position and says something like, "I was stressed out, off my meds, tired from the kids. I'm sorry." And then they make up and go back to playing their original roles.

Although each person gets to move among all the roles, one will often fit more comfortably in one role than in another based on personality, upbringing, and learned ways of coping. Here we overlap with topics we've discussed previously—managing anxiety and what you can't do. The rescuer, for example, was often an only child, or the oldest, or grew up in a chaotic family. He usually did not have many buffers between him and his parents and learned early on that he could avoid getting in trouble and avoid conflict by being good: "If I can stay on my toes and just do what my parents (and the teacher) want me to do all the time, I won't get in any hot water."

As a result, this type of person learns to be very sensitive to others as a means of survival and can pick up the nuances of emotions. But he is also ever-anxious, ever-ready to do what the parents want. Essentially, he says, "I'm happy if you're happy, and I need to make sure you are happy." And he gets rewarded for being good, and his head is filled with shoulds. What this person can't do is handle confrontation and strong emotions.

But what works for the child doesn't necessarily work so well for the adult. Now the world is bigger. Rather than just two or three important people to pay attention to, the rescuer adult has many more—the boss, the president of the local Rotary Club, the church minister. He now feels pulled in many directions, stretched thin, as he scrambles to accommodate what he thinks others want from him. He is overresponsible, easily feels like a martyr, and persists in the magical thinking that if he just does everything "right," others will somehow know what he needs and give it to him.

He also has a hard time knowing what he wants. Because he spent so much of his energy as a child looking outward and doing what others wanted, he never had the opportunity to sit back and decide what he wanted. Unlike following shoulds and rules, wanting is a feeling, and he is often unaware of what he is feeling. As an adult, if you ask him, "But what do you want?" he hesitates and gets stuck. He worries about making the right decision, not offending anyone in his life or that always-running critical voice in his head. Finally, a by-product of all this overresponsibility, of doing everything, is that the rescuer has gained control, and the control helps manage his anxiety. While he may define his control as "just getting others to do what makes sense" or "stepping up and helping out," others may see it for what it is—control—fueling the rescuer's feelings of being underappreciated.

Eventually, this holding in and walking on eggshells backs up and leads to burnout, depression, or shifting to the persecutor role. Because this creates so much drama and conflict, his worst dream coming true, he starts to shove it all back down again, only to have it build up. Wash, rinse, repeat.

The victim, in contrast, was often the youngest in the family, was abused or overprotected as a child by the parents, or had older siblings who stepped in and took over all the time when he was stuck with a problem. Just as the rescuer never learned to develop that gut sense of want or ability to handle confrontation, the victim never had opportunities to build the self-confidence that comes from learning to manage issues independently. As an adult, he quickly gets overwhelmed, underconfident, anxious. To handle these feelings, he looks to the rescuer, who takes over and helps him feel better.

Although most folks settle into rescuer or victim roles, there are some whose primary role is the persecutor and, in many ways, they are the rescuer's evil twin. While the rescuer's control is colored by being good and nice, the persecutor exercises control by being angry, critical, and blaming. This is the abuser, the school bully, the narcissistic personality. Often the persecutor's need to control is also driven by anxiety and hypervigilance: When I get scared, I get tough; if I can negatively control everything going on around me, no one can sneak up behind me and get me. For some, it is narcissism—others are objects to manipulate for personal gain; there's no empathy; there's a learned view of the world that there is me . . . and I take care of me.

This explains the dynamics of the triangle. But there's more—if we refer back to our diagram (page 54), you'll notice the two A's off to the side. Each A represents our Bowen's adult. Unlike the letters in the triangle, the A is not in a role; this is a complete person who is proactive rather than reactive, self-responsible rather than blaming; he lives outside the triangle. And the A's are peers; they are on the same level in terms of power; there is no one-up, one-down. This is where you want to be.

The adult says, "I'm responsible for what I think, do, say. If something bothers me, it is *my* problem. If you can do something to help me with *my* problem, I need to tell you, because you can't read my mind. If you decide not to help me, I'll need to decide what I will do next to fix my problem. Similarly, if something bothers you, it is *your* problem. That doesn't mean that I don't care, but if I can do something to help you with your problem, you need to tell me. And if I decide not to help you with *your* problem for some reason, you can work it out. You may not handle it the way I might, but you can do it. I don't need to take over."

There are two problems the rescuer and victim have in their relationship: one is that they expect a lot of mind reading—you should know what is going on or how to help without my having to say so—and then they feel frustrated and disappointed or angry when the other does not do it. The second is they also have a distorted sense of responsibility: The rescuer tends to be overresponsible because your problems are my problems; the victim tends to be underresponsible—my problems are your problems.

The adults, in contrast, are clear about who has the problem, represented by the vertical line running between them. If you feel it—your problem, your reaction—it's yours. This is a crucial concept, one invaluable for couples and individuals to understand and incorporate. This is Bowen's adult, and is also Al-Anon's approach to codependency. By being aware of who has the problem, the individuals can step back, take a deep breath, and avoid defensiveness, anxiety, taking control, and feelings of manipulation.

And for couples, this stance allows for intimacy. The rescuer's and victim's problem in their relationship is that the confines of their roles keep them stuck. The rescuer cannot let down his guard or get too vulnerable because he is afraid that the victim will not be able to manage. Similarly, the victim cannot ever get too strong because the rescuer will feel threatened and be out of a job. The line between the victim and rescuer within the triangle represents the emotional distance separating them.

The adults don't have this problem. Both can be responsible and strong, yet honest and vulnerable. They can take risks, are not locked in roles, and be more open and intimate. They are peers, represented by the horizontal line.

Two people can be in this pattern for a long time—seemingly getting along, suddenly having some acting out or emotional explosion, making up, returning to their roles, and repeating the pattern over and over again. Sometimes, particularly for the rescuer, the pattern will continue until he eventually drops from the weight of it all—he has a heart attack or a psychological breakdown, and everyone is surprised and afraid. What can also happen over time, which often brings the couple into therapy, is that one person is either tired of going around the cycle or begins to outgrow his role. Like any other pattern, it takes two to play the game, and as soon as one person begins to move toward the adult, the other gets scared and tries to pull him back in to keep the cycle going.

For example, you may have a rescuer who gets tired of being the martyr, of mopping up all the time; he starts to pull away and better define boundaries and problems. The classic case of this relationship is the codependent partner of an alcoholic. The wife, for example, begins to attend Al-Anon meetings and tells her husband, "I'm not going to call up your boss for you on Monday morning and tell him you are sick. You can call him yourself. I'm not going to pick you up off the front lawn on Saturday night if you get drunk." The partner is stepping out of the triangle, and if her husband regularly got drunk before, he will likely get rip-roaring drunk on Saturday night to try to hook her back into her former role. If that doesn't work, he is likely to switch to one of the other roles: He may shift to P—get angry and threaten to divorce her and get custody of the kids or cut off the money. Or he may shift to R—get nice, tell her how he will start attending AA meetings to appease her and bring her back.

Similarly, the rescuer feels threatened if the victim wants to move to the adult position. This is what I've often seen in the empty-nest stage of marriage. One partner has been more or less in charge—making most of the big decisions, financially supporting the family—and the kids begin to leave home. The other starts to say, "You know, I'm thinking of maybe going back to school. I never finished my degree because I stayed home with the kids, and now is a good time to do it; maybe I'll go back into full-time work; I think I'd like to get a checking and savings account so I can have my own money and be more independent."

While the more dominant partner knows what to do when the other is in the one-down position, he doesn't know what to do when roles shift. Generally, the first thing he will do is be nice but try to talk the less-dominant partner out of the changes: "Why do you want to go back to school now? You're 45 years old. What are you going to be able to do with a degree? It will cost us 60 grand for tuition; for what? You don't need to get a full-time job. This is a time to take it easy." Or "We don't need another checking account. It costs ten dollars a month in fees we don't need to spend." Stay put is the message. If that doesn't work, he may shift to the persecutor role and get angry—"If you want to go to school, you find a way to pay for it; we're not taking it out of our retirement." Or the dominant partner could move to the victim position and get depressed, so the other partner needs to care for him.

We also see this dynamic frequently in abusive relationships. Suppose the victim of a persecutor–victim relationship decides to move out of the triangle or out of the relationship and not be a punching bag anymore. In that case, the first thing the persecutor will do is more of the same. If he was angry, he is now going to get explosive. He will stalk her, hunt her down, emotionally abuse her or beat her up. If that doesn't work, he may get nice. He will call you for anger management because his partner thinks he has a problem. He may set up an appointment, but then, just as you're about to hang up, ask if you could do him a favor and phone his wife or girlfriend and let her know that he called about therapy; he'll never come for the first appointment, or ask then to let his partner know that he came, but then not follow through. If being nice doesn't work, he may get depressed and even threaten to kill himself so she will come back into the relationship.

If all the jockeying around fails, the person left behind has one of two choices. She may end the relationship and find someone else to play the corresponding role, someone to control and punish. Or the person left behind can move toward the adult position too.

The challenges of both partners moving to the adult position are several. The natural feeling of the one left behind is that if you care, you'll stay in the triangle. If they both move, the partners need to develop new ways of showing that they care for each other. There will be a transition period while these new ways are being created, and the new ways will not, at least for a while, feel as good as the old ones. There are also the challenges of learning new skills, especially for the partner left behind.

The triangle is so strong and continues for so long because, like most intimate relationships, the roles are complementary. Each sees in the other what he is unable to see in himself. The rescuer, for example, is not as nice or as strong as he thinks but sees his vulnerability and anger in the victim and persecutor. The victim is not as weak as he thinks but projects his strength and anger onto the rescuer and persecutor. The persecutor is not as tough as he thinks but only sees his weakness and goodness in the victim and rescuer.

By keeping this relationship triangle in mind as you talk with individuals or couples, you have a powerful assessment tool and a treatment map. By showing it to them, you can help them understand why they have those periodic blowups and acting-out behaviors—the affairs, the binge drinking, the shopping splurge. It also tells you, and them, what to move toward. Like the "standard" of Bowen's adult, like "what can't they do," you point out the gaps and the path to closing them. The rescuer needs to learn to recognize his wants and risk not being good and overresponsible. He needs to learn how to recognize his anger and use it for information about what he wants. He needs to experiment with letting go of control and resist the impulse to fix his anxiety by taking over when the other is struggling. He needs to learn how to let down his guard, to learn to trust and be vulnerable and nurture in a genuine caring way, rather than out of fear and the need for control.

Similarly, the victim needs to build up his self-confidence—by taking risks and doing things on his own, by using the rescuer not as a rescuer but as a support. He needs to learn how to partialize problems, so he doesn't feel overwhelmed. Like the rescuer, he needs to better tap into his anger and define his boundaries and wants.

Finally, the abuser needs to recognize that his anger is a defense. He has to look for the softer emotions in the victim—the hurt, the sadness, the regret—in himself and beneath the cover of his anger. He also needs to think about his strength as something that is more generous, needs to find ways of being nurturing and of allowing himself to be nurtured by the other.

Ways of Viewing Anxiety and Depression

Clients prone to anxiety and depression are in the victim role and have two voices in their heads: one that is telling them what they should do—the rescuer role—and the other that beats them up when they don't. Your goal is to help them move out of their depressed and anxious brain and into their rational one. Here you can help them check in with themselves and ask, "What voice is talking to me now? I'm going down the rabbit hole of anxiety with its 'what-ifs.' My depression is taking over, telling me, 'Why bother?' My critical voice tells me that I'm a loser and need to be more perfect and stop screwing up."

By being more aware of when the emotional brain is online, they can switch to the rational one. This is a skill you can demonstrate and teach in sessions and include in homework.

Parenting

The triangle can also describe the developmental relationship between parent and child. Children are, by default, dependent on their parents—in the V position. Parents are the R's. This makes sense—the child needs to lean on the parents for safety and skill building. But as children become adolescents, they become counterdependent: You say black because I say white; they vacillate between the one-down victim role to moving toward the adult role. Leave me alone and get off my back, versus I'm upset because I just broke up with my boyfriend. Here is where parents struggle—should I treat her as an adult or as a child? What is my role?

This is a difficult process. I've had to go through this with my own adult children, and the transition usually takes many years to work out. I've met thousands of 30-year-olds who are sensitive to their parents micromanaging their lives and treating them like ten-year-olds; often they rebel and act like fifteen-year-olds, some cutting their parents off for a few years. The challenge and the goal are to eventually shift the relationship from R/V to A/A.

Supervision

Finally, this model often describes the supervisor–supervisee relationship as it does the parent–child one. The similarities are apparent: the supervisee leans on the supervisor but eventually outgrows the relationship and wants to move toward the adult—to define her clinical style, to feel less micromanaged. This is what happened with Freud and Jung. Jung started pulling away and formulating his own ideas about development and archetypes, moving toward the adult; Freud couldn't cope with Jung's decision. He couldn't shift from teacher/rescuer to adult/adult. Freud ended the relationship, unable to handle the transition.

All this is a handy tool, whether you use it to assess why partners periodically have big fights or have affairs; why individuals always feel like the martyr, victim, or persecutor; why teens rebel with mixed messages; or why supervisees become restless and seem dismissive of your advice. It helps us remain clear about relationship dynamics, normal evolutions, and how personality shapes people's roles.

Think about how this may apply to your clients, but most important, to you. See what resonates and helps you see your relationship and clients differently and provides you with new ways of helping clients view themselves and their relationships.

CHAPTER 12

Making the Most of Parallel Process

I once supervised a team of therapists, most of them new grads, who did home-based work with families. The focus was usually on helping the parents create more structure by setting up rules and routines—a logical antidote to reining in the seemingly chaotic environment and helping their children feel less anxious. One common homework assignment was creating a reward chart for their children for doing homework, chores, or other tasks. The therapist would describe this chart to the parents, help them set it up, and suggest they use it during the week. The following week, the therapist would ask how the charting went and find that the parents hadn't used it. So the therapist and parents would walk through the process again; the parents would agree, but the next week the results were the same—no charting. By this point, some of the therapists would be frustrated. They would come down hard on the parents, grouse about how they were already in trouble with social services, that the parents needed to turn this around, that they, the clinicians, were there to help, and that the parents needed to get with the program—all understandable.

But scolding the parents was the worst thing they could do. Why? Because they weren't considering the parallel process.

The Anatomy of Parallel Process

You probably learned about parallel process at some point. Still, even if you didn't, you are undoubtedly familiar with it in everyday life: Sara is criticized by her boss, comes home, finds the house a mess, and her husband is watching television. She yells at her husband, who then yells at the kids, who then start fighting with each other. This is about emotions going down the line. And if we go back to our home-based work case, we can represent it with this diagram:

S ———————— T

T ———————— P

P ———————— C

What we have are parallel relationships. The S stands for supervisor, T for therapist, P for parents, and C for children, but we could just as easily substitute a partner. Starting at the bottom, we can track emotions going up the line. The children are not listening to the parents, the parents are frustrated and ignoring the therapist, and the therapist becomes frustrated with the parents. Showing his frustration and scolding the parents will likely get passed down, with the parents next scolding the children, which is only replicating what they probably always do.

As the clinician, you want to be aware of this process and be the one to stop and then change the emotional flow and climate rather than unconsciously recreate it. Even though you may feel frustrated, you need to step back, take a deep breath, override your impulses, and make that conscious clinical decision to treat the parents the way the parents need to treat the children. Rather than scolding, you need to be gentle, show empathy, and give support so the parents can learn to do the same.

If you don't, you will likely carry those emotions further up the line to your supervisor, replaying the parents' frustration and your own. This is similar to your partner complaining about how a customer treated him and, in describing what happened, actually replays how the customer sounded to him. Your supervisor needs to stop the emotional buck and treat you the way you need to treat the parents—not by scolding you about what you should have done, but with empathic and supportive listening. This is subtle but powerful.

Finally, we can bump this up one or two steps higher and imagine your supervisor passing those emotions further up the line instead of stopping the process. One common outcome of passing the emotional buck is the creation of a crisis-driven agency. Clients in crisis create a crisis in the staff that moves up the chain to the point where the director is overreacting to what has unfolded below. But sometimes, the crisis can start at the top and flow down. The agency director is panicking about funding. He rails at his program directors to focus on billing; your supervisor does the same in the next staff meeting, and now clinicians are hounding clients to pay their bills. Again, a crisis-driven, negative agency climate is created.

Here you may have little opportunity to change what is swirling around you, but you have an awareness of the process, which is always invaluable. This awareness can help you not get pulled into the larger culture or help you not unconsciously pass it down. At some point, you may realize that you need to push back and say what you need rather than taking what you get or, if necessary, decide that the workplace is not a good fit.

Parallel Statements

In addition to seeing how emotions go up and down the line, you can also look for parallel statements. Karen is complaining in sessions about how her mother always seems irritable. When you ask why she thinks her mother is that way, she pauses and then says that her mother probably is always stressed because she doesn't get enough support from Karen's father, and then pauses again and says that her father probably doesn't feel that he gets much support. Now Karen may be right. But if you hear this as a theme—if Karen essentially sees that the relationships around her are uncaring, unsupported—you might also wonder where this explanation is coming from: Out of all the things Karen could say, why is she saying this? Is she perhaps projecting her own feelings onto them? And the bigger question is, is she possibly feeling that you're not being supportive of her?

This is not an a-ha, figured-it-out, Dr. Freud truth, but rather something to explore. So you talk about ways Karen can be more supportive of her mother rather than becoming irritable around her to stop the emotional flow. But in the next session, you might say: "I noticed last week when you were talking about your parents that you said you thought they felt unsupported. I've also noticed that you said the same thing about others in your life. I'm just wondering, do you ever think I'm not supportive enough sometimes?" And you say this in a gentle voice.

Karen may say emphatically, "Absolutely not!" Or she may waver and then say, "Sometimes, but I realize that you have a demanding job, and it must be difficult to be empathic all day with everyone." Or she may say more clearly that yes, she often feels that you're good at problem solving but that she sometimes feels you don't take the time to listen and feels dismissed. Or she may say no, she's fine, and change the topic. Regardless of Karen's response, you put your concerns on the table. You're using your awareness of the parallel process to assess the state of the therapeutic relationship. You're also modeling how she might talk with her mother and repair a possible tear in your relationship with the client.

Being aware of and using the parallel process as information is yet another skill set, like listening for transference cues, that you may want to add to your toolbox. Start by keeping the diagram in mind when a client is talking about a problem in a relationship. Next, notice whether the client may be emotionally replicating the process and, if it appears so, tell yourself that you need to treat the client right now the way they ideally need to treat the other person. Usually, this means being compassionate and supportive, listening more, talking less, and giving the client room to vent. Rather than telling the client how to be, be that way in the room. See yourself as the dam that stops the emotional flow and reverses its course. And when you begin to hear themes in the client's relationship world, take the risk of turning the corner and ask if the client ever feels the same in their relationship with you.

And like all skills, mastering this one is a matter of practice. As suggested earlier, if you feel overwhelmed with too much to learn and practice, pick one or two skills to focus on, say in the next week or two, and ignore the rest. You don't have to do it all. You're building your clinical foundation in layers. And treat yourself the way you want clients to treat themselves—with patience and compassion.

CHAPTER 13

Shifting Focus

How Therapy Is Different from Normal Conversation

Just as you have a variety of clinical lenses to help clients view their problems, their world, and ultimately themselves in new ways, you also have additional lenses through which you can track and shape what is unfolding within the session process. This tracking and shaping is what makes therapy different from any other conversation; what makes the doing of therapy, therapy. In everyday conversations with friends and family, you're focusing on content, maybe at times emotions, but you're usually a passenger carried along by the conversational flow. During a therapy session, you are not only purposeful—moving through a specific agenda or toward a particular goal—but you are more alert, constantly monitoring and shifting your attention as you do. One moment, you are tracking Kate's medical history, but then you're noticing how she suddenly looks sad or shuts down or changes topics.

This ability to be in charge and calm while also being a bit hyperalert, scanning what is happening in the room, and quickly shifting focus is a bit like driving a car—watching the road, steering the wheel, looking in the mirror, and turning on signals while changing stations on the radio. This multilevel viewing and responding is its own skill set that, like learning to drive, can all seem overwhelming when starting out.

As with driving a car and the other multitask skill sets we've discussed, it helps to break them down. Here are some of the most common lenses you want to develop and use.

Content

We've talked about this already—that content generally fills clients' inboxes, what is easy for them and you to get lost within. To be clear, content is always essential, especially at the beginning of treatment. By talking about facts and figures, clients are constructing for you the current state of their lives—their emotions, struggles, and problems. You want to hear about them to understand where they are coming from, their own view of the world. What they present is what they want you to fix; this is about building rapport.

But this is where the conversation moves to therapy, and you shift from being the interested listener who wants to help keep the conversation going to the therapist, shaping the conversation for a purpose. So here you track: I'm getting confused. Did you go into the hospital once or many times? Are you currently taking medication, or have you stopped? You started therapy before but then dropped out—I don't understand why. Or you fill in the holes in your thinking: When you argue, how do you stop? When you feel anxious, where do you feel it most? Do you worry; do you have physical symptoms? When your father died, how did you handle it? You're connecting the dots, gathering the information you need to formulate a diagnosis and to develop a preliminary treatment plan.

Process

But at some point, you need to shift your focus—away from the facts of the story toward what is unfolding in the room. Jalen is getting teary; Jake pulls back in his chair, crossing his arms and shutting down. There's a problem in the room: the temperature rises or lowers; there's tension; your brilliant interpretation has been countered with a yes-but. You and the client have fallen out of step. In an everyday conversation, most folks just repeat what they've said, push harder, heap on more facts to make their case. But you don't do that. Content is now on the back burner. The new problem in the room is the emotion. You say to Jalen that she seems sad, and you say you wonder what just happened; you say that you notice Jake has pulled back and are wondering how he is feeling; you resist the urge to press your interpretation but instead say that it seems like they are thinking about this differently.

And what also makes this therapy is that you pay attention to yourself in this process. You are intentionally gentle in voice and posture with Jalen and Jake so they don't feel criticized and withdraw even more. Fix feelings with feelings, not facts, so you don't add fuel to the fire and actively begin to change the climate. Notice, decide on your focus, choose how to approach, then approach.

Third Ear

Third ear now seems old-school—shifting focus, slowing down for a few beats, and assessing what has unfolded in the past five to ten minutes. You realize that you've rambled on—giving a mini-lecture about anxiety—and probably overloaded your client with too much information. Or you've been asking many back-to-back questions and wonder if the client is beginning to feel interrogated. Or you realize you are shutting down because you're feeling overwhelmed by the couple's argument or flooded by too much backstory.

This is about process, but more about you in the process. Are you getting anxious? Is some countertransference kicking in that is shutting you down? Are you talking too much and interrupting rather than listening? Are you getting lost in the details of content?

If you don't know what to say, say you don't know what to say. Say that you realize you've been rambling, that you've probably dumped too much information on them, been asking too many questions, or feel a bit overwhelmed by their backstory. Check in with them, see where they are. Time to take the pulse of the session, to regroup. Like learning to steer the car, you're tweaking the process to keep the conversational car in the center of the lane.

Imagination

If we were to think of these different foci like rungs on a ladder, content might be at the bottom, with process and third ear next up, and at the top is this one: imagination. If tracking content, and even process, is like sniffing a trail like a bloodhound, this is where you follow no trail at all. Here you're mentally free-floating, paying attention to what images or memories are popping up in your head as the client is talking. Ruel is talking about his current state of unemployment and feeling isolated. You remember that summer years ago when you too were suddenly jobless or had an image of him standing alone in a large, empty room.

Certainly, this is about you, but that doesn't mean it's something you need to ignore. It's your unconscious and past coming to the surface. Sharing them—briefly telling Ruel about your summer and the similar feelings you had or that image of the room—can be unexpectedly powerful. It also introduces and models the notion of stream of consciousness into the therapy process. Ruel may find himself straying from the long trail of facts and being more open to his memories and images.

What to Do

Like learning to drive the car, shifting focus like this is about creating new pathways in your brain, heightening your senses. At first, you want to do this deliberately—reminding yourself before the start of a session to check in on these different levels—perhaps knowing what informational content you need or intentionally shifting focus to take the temperature of the room, periodically seeing who is engaged, who is pulling back, taking a few deep breaths, and checking in with your third ear.

But also step back and assess your strengths and weaknesses. For example, you may be limber with individuals but can get too caught up in content when seeing a couple or family. Or you realize that angry men trigger your countertransference, and it's easy for you to freeze and miss what is unfolding. You'll want to bring up this issue with your supervisor to unravel or role-play, or perhaps have a cotherapist for those couple or family sessions—so you don't feel the pressure of having to do it all—to help you focus on process while your colleague handles content.

Finally, you can practice shifting focus outside of the therapy session. For example, don't play therapist when having lunch with a friend, but experiment and practice your shifting lenses in a more relaxed atmosphere.

If you know how to drive, skate, and play an instrument, you already know the art of shifting focus, and undoubtedly you already have a pretty good base to start from. Like those other skills, practice will make your ability to shift focus smoother and more natural.

Practice and be patient.

CHAPTER 14

Therapy's Many Voices

In the last chapter, we discussed how therapy differs from everyday conversation. Here we're taking a step back and looking at the larger landscape: What are we doing when we're doing therapy? Obviously, it depends partly on your clinical model, whether you focus on unraveling the past, looking for patterns in current relationships, or teaching skills—all effective approaches for helping clients solve their presenting problems. But we can also look at what we offer clients in terms of what I call our many voices. Here are some of the most common ones that come to mind.

Voice of Reason

Although Harry admits that his boss is a nice guy, he still worries that if he voices any complaints about his work schedule, his boss might fire him. Sherry can't help thinking that even though she has been with her boyfriend a long time, it's only a matter of time before he gets tired of her and leaves. Angelo has been laid off from his job and spends the day binge-watching on YouTube. Ask him why he's not been applying for jobs; he says there's no sense looking for one—no one will hire him.

Clients develop distorted, irrational thinking for a lot of good reasons. We can imagine that Harry has a generalized anxiety disorder, and his anxious brain is constantly creating worst-case scenarios. Or Sherry may have a history of trauma or a long string of breakups that leave her wired for eventual disaster. Angelo is likely depressed after being laid off. In his depressed state, he understandably is cynical or self-critical or adapts the "Why bother? It doesn't matter" attitude that comes with depression.

When a client's rational brain is off-line, and the emotional brain runs the show due to anxiety, trauma, and depression, you become the rational brain. Here you can walk Harry through his thinking: Despite his being a nice guy, does his boss also have a temper, is he an autocrat, has he eliminated others who have spoken up? By asking these questions, you're that voice of reason, and you're also finding out how his mind works, where he emotionally gets stuck, and you can do the same with Sherry and Angelo. You may choose to take the educational route and talk about the effects of anxiety, trauma, and depression on the brain, or go historical and explore similar situations from their pasts that may fuel their current thinking. Whatever option you pick, you are challenging their assumptions and worldview; by doing so, they can begin to do the same.

Voice of Reality

I once saw a mom who had lost custody of her two sons when they were elementary school age. The boys lived close by. She would drive by their house periodically and see them playing outside; she would wave, and they would turn their backs. She sent letters, emails, and birthday cards, never receiving a reply or an acknowledgment. Although she remained single, she always rented a two-bedroom apartment that she struggled to afford; the second bedroom, she said, was for the boys. She believed, hoped, and imagined that as the boys moved into their teen years, they would one day show up at her door and ask to be taken in. Could this happen? Perhaps, but clearly, it was a long shot, and like Harry, Sherry, and Angelo, there seemed to be distorted thinking at play, driven perhaps by trauma or grief, magical thinking, or denial.

The labels don't matter, and while I tried to be that voice of reason—aligning the facts in ways that were different from hers, this was also about facing limits, the voice of reality. Despite her outreach over the years and doing the best she could, she couldn't control the outcome or what her children would do or think. Clients struggle with situations like this all the time: needing to realize that what they believe is a problem may not be a problem to someone else; clashing with others over means and losing sight of ends; or although it seems that they have no options, they have many options, however difficult they may be. Being the voice of reality is helping clients see their world not through the *real* lens but a different one, becoming clear about their choices and limits.

Voice of Change

And change is another powerful voice. Harry speaks up and talks to his boss; the mom accepts the reality of her situation and moves to a one-bedroom apartment. The change is evident, but often, it is not. We all can have tunnel vision in our lives; incremental changes are difficult for us to notice; they lack the clarity of, say, physical rehab where you realize you walked further today than you did a few days ago. Sherry has a wisp of recognition that her boyfriend's seeming quietness does not only trigger the vague anxiety she has been feeling the last day or so, but probably triggers some stirring of an old wound. But still, it is a wisp that fades so quickly that it is barely noticed and seen as some aberration.

Here's where you step in. You notice and chronicle changes that the client can't see—that they sound and are more assertive or less self-critical or are able to rein in those strong emotions more quickly than before. You notice, label, and emotionally get out the balloons and confetti to celebrate their movement. You help them see what they yet cannot.

Voice of Clarity

Here we're talking about asking the hard questions, cutting to the chase. The couple volleys complaints at each other and agrees that this pattern has been going on for years. You ask, "How bad is this? Are you thinking about divorce?" Or ask the parents of a drug-addicted child if they ever feel like they should have seen the signs and symptoms earlier or done something differently. Or you ask the client who says he has an "anger problem," just like his father, why he doesn't do more to rein it in.

This is not about accusation, criticism, or judgment but about normalizing, diagnosing, or simply digging deeper. This is about talking about the elephant in the room, about saying what you suspect the client or clients have already been thinking and, by doing so, getting things on the table, or reassuring them that this thinking and doing is understandable. Or by asking the hard questions, making a strong statement, they, in turn, become more clear themselves: No, we would never consider divorce, say each of the partners; no, we did the best we could, say the parents, considering how frightened we were; yes, I didn't think I was making excuses for my anger, but hearing you ask that, I realize I was, just as my father did. By being bold in the unfolding process, clients can do the same.

Voice of Accountability

Angelo agrees to apply to three jobs this week; Sherry is willing to have a serious "state of the union" conversation with her boyfriend to help her feel more secure. And then you follow up—did you do it, what happened; if not, why not, what got in the way? This is about moving clients along on a path of change; knowing that you will ask them the following week if they did their homework and will nudge them to do it. You're not the scolding mommy or daddy but the sideline coach working with the client to tackle the problem.

Voice of Compassion and Hope

This, of course, is what we do most: offering compassion so clients are not alone with their pain, offering hope that change is possible despite their overwhelming feeling that they will never change. The grief will subside; if you speak up, your partner may be upset, but now conversations can be more honest and problems have a better chance of being resolved; that there truly is light at the end of the tunnel even if we don't know the ultimate outcome; by doing the best you can do, you are doing the best you can do, and that's good enough.

Obviously, there is a theme connecting these different voices—you're offering clients new perspectives, new lenses through which to view themselves and others to replace the old, worn-out ones that no longer work and leave them feeling stuck. It speaks to the different roles we therapists can take—advocate, compassionate supporter, challenger—and literally different voices—bold, assertive, curious, empathetic. Like other tools, you can decide when and how to use them in your clinical toolbox.

But these voices often represent not so much our therapeutic skills but our place outside the client's world. Unlike family or friends who not only have their own views of the client honed from shared experiences, we do not. Unlike them, who may be cautious about saying what they think, we can afford to be bold. And most of all, as outsiders, we can see the bigger picture and the blind spots that the client can't recognize.

Voice of You

But wait, there's one more voice that is less about technique and about being deliberate and more about a way your clients can solidify the gains they have made. It can also be an unexpected gift to you. It happens when clients, who are often in longer-term therapy but sometimes (surprisingly) after a few sessions, begin to talk about you as part of their thought process: "So I had the situation come up with ____________ and I said to myself, 'What would you do?' And I thought about it and decided to do ____________." Your client has begun not only to hear what you say, but also to internalize what you say, how you think, how to act differently. The client is starting unconsciously to use you as a role model, undoubtedly so different from all the other role models she has had in her life.

This is a gift, in that you realize that you are making an impact often despite your perceptions. During those hard times and hard days, knowing how you are making a difference can be enough to keep you going.

So, here's some homework: Think about which of these voices you are comfortable with, and which of them you are less so. Next, be curious and experiment with incorporating those less-comfortable ones into your sessions to see what effects they have on the process and can eventually become part of your clinical repertoire.

CHAPTER 15

Therapy as a Pragmatic Sport

Even your family doctor doesn't get it right all the time. Her prescription for your rash didn't help; the antibiotic wasn't strong enough; she tried something else or referred you to a specialist. Medicine is trial and error. Antonio Machado suggests, "Traveler, there is no path. The path is made by walking" (Berg & Maloney, 2003).

Therapy too is a pragmatic sport, not one for the perfectionistic or rigid, nor the impulsive or reckless. Here are some guidelines to help you create and walk the middle path.

Determine Criteria for Progress

This is a front-end decision based on the client's goals and your own. Jake wants to stop snapping at his kids or be less obsessive about cleaning his apartment. In collaboration with Jake, your treatment plan pins down what "cleaning his apartment" looks like. But Jake also admits that while he's tried therapy before, the most he's ever completed is a few sessions. So, continuing to show up rather than drop out becomes a goal and a criteria for progress.

What you don't want to do is have vague, undefined measures for success. Coming every week can easily lapse into dependency, in which there is seeming motivation and a good therapeutic relationship, but you and the client are treading water. Doing those regular check-ins to step back and assess the state of treatment is a good way to prevent dependency from happening.

That said, you may have long-term clients for whom showing up is the treatment and goal. Ellen, for example, has a many-year history of mental illness, and she comes every week for support and accountability—check-ins to see how she is managing and whether she is taking her medications. Without this regular contact, Ellen can go off her meds, go downhill quickly, and wind up in the state hospital or on the streets. The criteria for progress, in this case, is holding steady.

Don't Confuse Means and Ends

When doing couple or family therapy, it's easy for partners or family members to resist, either because they don't believe there is a problem or often because they think that therapy is not the way to solve it. A conflict ensues in the session about therapy versus no therapy, and they look to you to be the judge. The step-back perspective and reality check here are about realizing and accepting that therapy is a means to solve problems and not an end; you want to focus on the ends.

Sixteen-year-old Nick and his mom come to their first appointment. The mom is worried that Nick's recreational drug use has turned into something more and is pushing him to have individual therapy. Nick agrees that maybe he does have a bit of a monkey on his back but digs in and refuses therapy.

"Okay," you say, "but what are you willing to do?"
"Try NA meetings."
"Great," you say. "Go for it and see if it helps."

Similarly, while it's clear to you that Tanya can benefit from treatment for her anxiety and depression, it's also equally clear that she doesn't have the psychological energy and time to devote to it. But she's willing to check out medication or join a more open-focused support group at her church, and that's a better path for her right now. Try it, you say. Again, it's about solving the problem rather than creating resistance by arguing over the means.

But this confusion of means and ends can snarl even everyday relationships: Carl and Aaron argue about what chores the kids should do, go back and forth about who is right, and in the process, lose sight of the purpose of doing chores at all. Or Amy, to "get healthy and develop better habits" becomes hyperfocused on an exercise plan or on doing meditation a certain way; she injures herself, gets frustrated with the meditation, and then beats herself up for quitting.

Here you help Carl, Aaron, and Amy step back and refocus on the ends, the goals they have lost sight of. You challenge them to stop the arguing or hyperfocusing by challenging them to brainstorm other options. This is not about chores, exercise, or meditation but about helping clients be less myopic, more flexible and creative. The danger is that you too get pulled into the weeds with your clients—helping them fine-tune the chore list or the exercise program. You too lose sight of the ultimate end.

Know the Limits of Your Skills

Whitney initially presented with depression and anxiety, but a few sessions in, she disclosed that she had been bingeing and purging for the last year. Or Kendall's "occasional" use of alcohol is not only increasing but has become the center of his days and weeks—he's sliding into addiction. You're not trained in treating eating disorders or addiction. Like your family doctor who realized she was out of her knowledge league when the second prescription didn't work, you've learned the same—time to call the cavalry. Depending on the client's need and your skills, getting help may involve consulting with a specialist, receiving intensive supervision, bringing in a cotherapist, or getting a second opinion. But the key is knowing and acknowledging the limits of your skills.

Realize When It's Time to Ramp Up

While knowing the limits of your skills tells you when to get help or stop, you also want to know the bottom lines with your clients in terms of their progress: Knowing when Whitney or Kendall don't just need a different focus and treatment plan but need to be in an inpatient setting for a few weeks. If you're not sure, talk with your supervisor or have a consult with a trusted colleague.

The theme here is that good therapy is about flexibility, adaptation, not getting stuck in a rut in process or in content, and being willing to think outside the box to reach goals. Regardless of the path an individual case may ultimately follow, this pragmatic approach is not just about therapy but about navigating life.

CHAPTER 16

Creative Formats

Thinking Outside the Box

When you think about doing outpatient therapy, what probably comes to mind are weekly sessions for some varying period of time. What determines how long you see a client, couple, or family? The top reason is likely your clinical model. If you use a psychodynamic approach rather than, say, a solution-focused one, not only does the latter usually have a built-in session cap that the former does not, but the model's goals themselves shape the treatment length.

But regardless of your model, the client's presenting problem will also be a factor. The client who is feeling suicidal or has an active eating disorder is not going to get much benefit from a few sessions. Nor is a family in chaos, with multiple issues on the front burner that they summarily dump in your lap. And then there's always the client's own expectations and needs. Clients who feel they need ongoing support to get them through those seemingly never-ending rough patches in their lives, or those who feel it is finally the time to dig out those still haunting ghosts of the past, are not going to be happy campers when you tell them you specialize in single-session therapy.

But in addition to all this clinical stuff is the nonclinical—your workplace or job description. Your agency may not follow a solution-focused approach, and budget, population, staffing, and mission limit treatment to ten sessions. Or you work in a walk-in crisis center where you see clients for one session or two at the most or in emergency services where your job is to take an hour or two to evaluate and then transfer patients to . . . somewhere.

Yet another factor determining how long you see clients is not your job setting or even your clinical model, but you—your willingness to entertain and experiment with different formats, your ability and willingness to think outside the box, be creative about how to do therapy. By imagining options to the session-a-week-for-a-TBD-period model, you are not only opening your practice to working with a broader range of clients and their needs, but you are expanding your skills and increasing your flexibility and self-confidence. And when you may begin to feel a bit bored and stale with your everyday everyday, having different ways of doing your job can make the difference you need.

So here I offer a few creative formats, not only as possibilities to consider, but also to help you think outside the box. See what grabs you.

Single Session/Brief Sessions/Limited Sessions

What can you do in a single session or in just a few sessions? Actually, a lot or at least enough. One-and-done or several-session models have been in place for several decades now, and the research shows that they are effective and that clients leave satisfied (Brown, Lambert, Jones, & Minami, 2005; Leichsenring, Rabung, & Leibing, 2004). In my own practice, I have had clients who came once and, despite my reaching out, never returned. But I'm no longer surprised when I find that I receive referrals of friends and family from many of these same folks, who laud their brief time with me.

Once any discussion about brief therapy gets under way, usually some skeptic will question whether coming for a few sessions actually leads to long-term change, change that sticks. My answer: Good question but a moot point. While some clients are seeking long-term therapy and perhaps even long-term change, my experience is that most are not. These one-time or brief therapy models work, I believe, because they provide what many clients are seeking—help with a specific problem or situation or taking the edge off their current crisis. Unlike going to the therapeutic equivalent of an orthodontist and knowing they are committing to years of weekly tweaking, they're going to the dentist with a toothache and are willing to plop themselves in a chair long enough to get the cavity filled and the pain stopped. Clients want to reduce the angst of that big argument on Saturday and get back to baseline, to have concrete ideas about how to talk to their teen this week about her drug use, or to better manage their social anxiety because they are bottoming out with loneliness or have a command performance coming up and are feeling overwhelmed.

We know from the research on habit formation that changing one central piece of a dysfunctional pattern—the keystone habit—ripples out, builds on its own momentum, and creates new functional ones (Duhigg, 2014): Eating more vegetables can lead to healthier eating overall, which can, in turn, lead to losing weight, that leads to starting exercise, that leads to quitting smoking—a behavioral Rube Goldberg device set in motion. Similarly, the conversation with the teen changes the family dynamic not because it is necessarily about drugs but because it is a different conversation—the parents are less accusatory and more honest—which helps the teen be the same, which in turn changes the family climate for the better, that then snowballs. Or armed with concrete conversational tips, the anxious client's not quite so nervous, a different and better experience unfolds, and the experience, in turn, makes risk taking easier, leading over time to less anxiety and greater self-confidence.

Who a Brief Model Is Good For

Clients seeking concrete advice and skills with a specific problem or situation—for example, the child throwing tantrums, the discovery of an affair, actors auditioning for a part. Those needing help making a decision—ending a relationship, taking a job, putting grandma in a nursing home.

Who a Brief Model Is Not Good For

Clients specifically seeking long-term or supportive therapy; those with complex issues, such as eating disorders, addictions, personality disorders, persistent trauma symptoms, and psychotic disorders, for example. Clients needing ongoing support—those with chronic mental health issues or with ongoing disabilities, such as an intellectual disability.

What to Do

- Clarify expectations; explain your model—one, two, or several sessions. You can discuss this option in a presession phone call or even explain this option on your website.
- Help the client(s) define specific goals—what, concretely, do they want to take away from the session(s)—so you both know what you are striving for.
- Take an active role. This is not a time to sit there, nod your head, and

ask, "How does that make you feel?" Keep the goal in mind; move forward.

- Give concrete suggestions and teach practical skills; use homework to help them move forward outside sessions.
- Consider spreading out sessions: Rather than seeing clients weekly, see them biweekly so they have more time to practice skills.

Intensives

Cindy's elderly parents are visiting for a week, and she wants to take advantage of the opportunity to schedule a couple of back-to-back sessions with her and her parents to resolve some long-standing issues; Alex has always had a fear of public speaking, has to make a major presentation next week, and is freaking out; Bill has to decide by the end of the week whether to take a lucrative job overseas; a couple who lives out of state has heard wonderful things about you and is willing to see you, but because of the time and distance, are hoping they can do several sessions over a long weekend.

Think of intensives as concentrated brief therapy, similar to the difference between attending a three-hour workshop and a three-day one. Clients still have time to address the problems under the problem, to learn skills, and to get the support they need to make that decision or begin to resolve that problem, but with a bit less depth or practice time.

Who an Intensive Model Is Good For

Clients who, for practical reasons such as time, distance, and logistics, want a concentrated dose of therapy. Also families, couples, or individuals in crisis who need therapeutic first aid or clients who need to make a major decision. This model is also often incorporated into residential treatment, where, for example, parents may come to a residential eating disorder center and engage in a series of educational and family sessions with their child on a long weekend to focus on resolving core family issues and gain information and insight that can be applied at home following discharge.

Who an Intensive Model Is Not Good For

Clients with complex issues needing long-term treatment. That said, this format can jump-start more extended treatment, for example, a several-session family intervention that enables the identified patient to begin residential treatment.

What to Do

- Like with other brief models, you need to have clear goals and take an active role.
- Same-day homework is helpful—for example, a couple may be given an exercise to do as individuals or together that evening, or an individual might work up a pro-and-con list for the new job, which becomes the focus for the next session.
- Most important, you need to step up, show leadership, and choreograph the time to maximize the experience and achieve your clients' goals. For example, if you are working with a couple or family, you may decide to see them together for a session, then see each person individually, and then bring them back together. You may have specific background information that you feel is essential to gather, topics to discuss, educational information to share, exercises that you want to build into the process to enhance the overall experience. Think of your role as providing more of a workshop than simply a series of sessions.

Virtual Residential

Virtual residential can seem like an odd duck in the therapy world. Virtual residential takes intensives to a deeper level and is usually used as an alternative to residential treatment. Here you are replicating the residential experience by offering therapy sessions daily or checking in with a client by phone, text, or Zoom several times a day. You actually end up spending several hours a day in the client's home providing a variety of treatment activities or working as part of a treatment team being available 24/7 in the event of crises. For example, this model may be fitting for clients who are severely depressed or struggling with addiction and ideally need residential treatment but, because of distance, money, availability, or resistance, cannot or will not attend. Or it could be suitable for those transitioning out of intensive therapy—clients just discharged from residential treatment for an eating disorder and who need steady support to prevent relapse or teens needing help acclimating back into family life or school after spending three months in residential treatment for addiction.

Although most of this work is offered by agencies specializing in such services, I've known colleagues who make such types of services their specialty.

Who Virtual Therapy Is Good For

Clients who need residential treatment but, for various reasons, it's not an option; those transitioning out of residential treatment.

Who Virtual Therapy Is Not Good For

Clients who are medically or emotionally unstable—who need containment for safety, or 24-hour monitoring, or need to be assessed for and stabilized on medication and require a residential or hospital setting.

What to Do

- Assess for appropriateness. You need to be able to rule out who is not appropriate for such a program at the start—for example, determining active suicidality versus severe depression, food restriction versus medical instability. Once virtual therapy is in place, you need to have clear markers of progress and clear criteria to decide when it is not working or is not practical and you need to change gears.
- Decide on the level of support. Does the client need a daily session, twice-daily check-ins, fewer sessions, or more? Generally, you start with the more intensive level and dial down as the client improves.
- Have a team. In these complex cases, you want a team of other professionals to support you and the client. For example, someone coming out of residential treatment for an eating disorder will usually need a combination of dieticians, therapists, psychiatrists, or group therapy—someone every day to help the client stay on track. If someone is struggling with addiction, it is much the same—daily contact with AA/NA or the client's sponsor or family members—so you are not doing this therapy alone.

So, have I piqued your interest? Better yet, have I stirred your creativity? When we look back at the history of our profession, every advancement in our field is the product of new and radical ideas that therapists were willing to try. Sigmund Freud decided to have clients lie down on a couch and say whatever came into their heads, while Harry Stack Sullivan would sit next to clients, staring straight ahead so they could both share the same emotional vision as they talked. Fritz Perls had folks talk to empty chairs, while Richard Schwartz has clients access their own internal source of healing energy.

You too can be such a pioneer. You too can think of unique new ways to see others, help others, treat others.

You just need to step out of your box.

CHAPTER 17

Therapy as Performance

Life may be a moment-by-moment experience, but as the mindfulness folks continually remind us, most of our moments are lost in a haze of routine and running on autopilot. One of the gifts of doing and receiving therapy is that for that short period of time, there is the opportunity to break out of that haze. In a session, there's a clear rather than scattered focus; there are no interruptions; clients are out of their routine. It's just you and her or you and them; life concentrated.

But therapy doesn't stop there. The foundations and tools of the therapy process itself can heighten that experience even further. Sessions can be, for many, a nonreligious confessional; for others, a sanctum of security: Here is the one place where I can say how I think and feel—my secrets, my sins, my past—and not be judged or worry that someone will be upset; here is where I can get advice without bias.

And even when you respond with textbook-style active listening—engaged but not interrupting, not jumping in with finger-wagging comments about what-you-should-do, what-were-you-thinking—the impact is often profound. Clients have discovered a place and a person that helps them relax, truly be themselves, and say what they're thinking, and by saying what they're thinking, they learn not only what they're thinking but who they are. This is the simple power of therapy—disclosing, and by disclosing, discovering.

The moral here is that therapy, even at its basic level, doesn't require much to be effective. But because good therapy is about shaping the experience that unfolds within a session—deciding how you'd like clients to feel differently today when they leave than when they came in—because it's always about human-on-human, because we are creatures of habit, there is always the danger of falling into a routine, a haze, the ordinary, of diluting its power. It happens, and on some days and sessions, that is fine—you both need a breather, a time to catch up and chat rather than dig. But if you worry that the "some days" can turn into a new norm, it's time to have more proactive tools in your toolbox that can help you create those corrective emotional experiences, ones that allow clients to view their lives and their past, present, and future in a new way.

Here are some suggestions; some you may know and can review, and others you may want to experiment with.

Reframing

"While I know you're feeling depressed and have emotionally been here before, this sounds different: Your mother has just died, and because you had to handle all that came with her passing, you said that you marched ahead, became the good soldier. What you're feeling now isn't about depression, but grief, your sense of loss, and loss follows a different script."

"Your daughter is struggling at school, and you are worried that she is just a bad kid who simply doesn't like school. But it seems like she may have an attention problem; she struggles to focus and stay still. She's not being bad; this is how her brain works."

"You say your husband doesn't want to go out, is not as active as he was when he was working, and I understand you are frustrated and see him as lazy. Retirement is difficult for many, especially those whose identity is tied to work. I think what understandably seems like him being lazy may be his struggling with a difficult but normal period of transition to retirement."

Just as your doctor tells you that that dark spot on your face is not the cancer you fear it is but the benign result of too many hours in the sun, you too are putting the client's worry and problem in a new light. You see and know what they cannot. By your viewing their situation in a new way, they can back out of that anxiety-driven rabbit hole they've been going down. You provide that reality check, and they feel better.

Defining Similarities to Counter Differences

Becca and William are replaying their last argument, which quickly dissolves into arguments about facts—who said what, when; they are caught up in their different realities. But what you hear most is that they are each saying the same thing—that they feel lonely, feel frustrated with problems they cannot solve, or are worried about their son. You say this: You both are arguing over facts but talking about the same thing differently. You both feel the same, you share the same problem; you are more alike than different.

Interpretations

Or Sue complains about her brother, a slacker, she says, who drives her crazy. You recall aloud how she said the same about her father. You wonder whether her brother reminds her of her father and that maybe this is fueling her reaction to him. This is the classic psychodynamic interpretation in which you help the client see how the past is being projected on and replayed in the present. It is about the brother, but not only the brother; it's also about the father. Like reframing and finding similarities, you offer a new lens, creating a new opportunity and approach.

Sculptures, Guided Imagery

Shaban and Eric are considering divorce, and you ask each of them to take turns sculpting their relationship as a sculptor might to represent how emotionally it feels to them. Shaban has them holding hands, but with each turned away. Eric places himself on his knees, looking up at Shaban as she points her index finger at him and has a scolding look on her face. Or you guide Jeff through a guided imagery exercise about his life—as a child, a teen, a young adult, and in the present—and at each age, he is alone, frightened, or angry.

Like dreams, these techniques create raw images that provide new information in a powerful way.

Role Plays

Bill wants to ask his supervisor about getting a raise but feels intimidated. You let Bill play his boss, and you, Bill. You model for him what he could say, how he could respond. You debrief and ask how he felt; you explain what you did and why, then let him practice what he might say with you. Role plays are "boots-on-the-ground" experiences that not only teach skills but reduce anxiety and increase self-confidence.

Educational Speeches

Much therapy is about teaching—for example, helping clients understand anxiety and depression or the behaviors of early I-hate-you teens. But as we already discussed, you can increase your impact by crafting powerful speeches. The key is crafting—carefully choosing your words and what to emphasize—and your body posture. Find role models by watching videos of movie speeches you admire to add power to your presentation. Practice in your mirror with your family.

Experience before Explanation

Learning and being comfortable with these techniques put you at the ready, but just as important is knowing the best time to deliver them. The rule of thumb is: experience before explanation. Here's what that means.

Let Clients Describe the Problem and Express Their Emotions

Here you reframe the child's possible attention problem only after the parents have described his school behavior and frustration. You talk about how each partner feels lonely after they both have expressed their loneliness. You invite them to do the sculpture, or the role play, and give your educational speech only after they have not only explained the situation, but you've been able to draw out and label their underlying emotions. Now that they feel heard, you have an opportune time to step in.

If you do this before the story is out or the emotions are expressed, the information is merely information; it lands on their rational brains. You want to maximize the experiential impact by generating and building on the emotional climate.

Launch the Experience without Explanation

Just as engaging your technique too quickly can kill the emotional experience, so can a preliminary explanation: "I'd like you to try this because . . . " followed by a long explanation. Don't do that. Instead, say "I'd like to try to do a role play—are you willing to do it?" Then do it.

Then Explain

After the experience, it's time to debrief so the client can get her rational brain back online, make sense of the experience, and leave without feeling rattled or upset. Your explanation at this point is grounding.

Your challenge: Think about how you can make your sessions more experiential. Take one or two techniques at a time and experiment with them. Plan them out ahead of time and then look for suitable openings. If you don't have enough time, don't try and squeeze them in at the end, but save them for next time. You are creating a repertoire of skills, learning to use other aspects of yourself, and enhancing your clinical impact. Try them, avoid being too self-critical, and be curious.

CHAPTER 18

Handling Self-Disclosure

There are a few big divides (practical and theoretical) in the world of therapy: Focus on the past versus the present; reflection and insight versus action and skills; long-term treatment versus short-term treatment. But an additional one is the issue of self-disclosure: How much do you share information about yourself with your clients? If your theoretical foundation is, say, psychoanalysis, the answer is simple: you don't; the therapist is a blank slate. But for most of us, it's an issue that doesn't have a simple answer. Self-disclosure is on a continuum from a tiny bit to a lot. Where you ultimately decide to land usually reflects some combination of theory and clinical style—your "use of self." If you are struggling with this question, I offer these guidelines.

Start with Your Clinical Theory

Having a theory to build upon provides ballast to your work. It is where you can return to recenter. It keeps you from drifting off into anxiety, from inventing the wheel with each new client and letting your personal "stuff" contaminate the therapeutic relationship. Even if your approach is somewhat eclectic—pulling on a bit of CBT, ACT, DBT, existential, solution-focused, object relations, whatever—it's still your model. Hopefully, you are clear not only on what and why you believe and do, but also that you use your theory to set and maintain your vision of what you think therapy is all about. Each theory carries a way of looking at the therapeutic relationship itself. How you see the relationship and your role will help you pick a starting point on the self-disclosure continuum.

Proactively Determine Your Own Boundaries

"Are you married?" "Do you have kids?" What's your comfort zone not about answering these specific questions but answering clients' questions overall? Develop your policy based on your theory and comfort level; map this out for yourself in advance so you don't have to stumble and think on your feet. Even more important, this mapping helps keep your countertransference with specific clients at bay.

Without clear guidelines, there's the danger of your sharing personal information based on your relationship with certain clients; the unevenness is a red flag for countertransference. Sharing can especially happen with longer-term clients. "And how was your week?" asks your client, and you're off and running, and chatter fills the therapeutic hour. Therapy dilutes into these chats, quasi-friend relationships, and dependency on both sides. Unless you have a solid clinical rationale for choosing to have such conversations, you're not doing therapy.

But at worse, it is worse. You're not diluting; you're distorting. There's a big difference between answering a client's question about whether you are married with a simple yes and saying to the same client who is struggling in his marriage that you too have had similar struggles. The difference is big, but the line between them is hair-width small. Again, this doesn't mean you would never talk about your marriage, but you're walking a tightrope between rationale and rationalization, and it's all too easy to slip.

Disclose Based on Clinical Need

Now I'm going to confuse you. Having a personal policy helps you not to stray into distorted therapeutic relationships. That said, self-disclosure is a powerful therapeutic tool. Here you may tell a teen a story about your struggle with high school cliques or how you learned to manage your anxiety at her age. You're deciding to tell the story to (1) normalize her experience, (2) humanize the way she may be seeing you and create rapport and a safe space, (3) deliberately take on the role of caring adult to offset the criticism or neglect she gets from other adults in her world, (4) offer her hope that her problems are solvable, or (5) all the above. You may do much of the same when talking to the client struggling in her relationship and commenting about how you moved through difficult times in your past relationships or sharing a brief history of your childhood trauma.

What's important is that your self-disclosure is clinically driven—not from emotionally based, ever-diluting professional boundaries but out of a clinical strategy. The all-of-the-above with your teen can, you believe, be psychologically potent—it is what she is missing in her life, and she feels isolated and different. You're not talking off the top of your head based on your reaction, but it is planned and paced. And you are clear in your mind about the purpose and point that you are trying to make, and you state this—so the client understands the context and takeaway, so there are no misunderstandings or reading into your disclosure.

Like a lot of therapy, deciding about the use of self-disclosure is a challenge: How much, when, with whom? When you feel the urge to speak up about yourself in the middle of a session, pause and ask yourself, Why this, why now, why with this particular client? Once again, this work is difficult (and rewarding) because it is person to person, and our humanness and desire to help and connect draw us in. The goals are to be intentional and deliberate, and if you are confused or uncertain, talk to your supervisor or a trusted colleague.

This is ultimately about creating your clinical style that allows you to be yourself and be yourself in service of the client.

CHAPTER 19

Sounds of Silence

Like poker players in a James Bond movie doing the blink contest as they try to read each other's tells, you and your client sit staring at each other. Or maybe you're not staring, but one of you has suddenly broken eye contact as though distracted by some stain on the rug. But no matter the heads or the eyes, what's most noticeable is the silence that stretches out throughout the room.

We each have our own relationship with silence, baked into our psychology—the introvert on a long plane flight has no problem ignoring his row mate, while the extrovert gets restless and talkative after a half hour. Or our physiology—the child with ADHD gets squirmy in class and begins playing with her pencil or elbowing the kid next to her rather than focusing on her worksheet. But silence is also woven into our family culture—the marked differences between those families who physically fill our offices but are verbally absent in stark contrast to those that are forever chattering even as they come down the hall. Or silence is woven into our ethnic or religious cultures. When visiting a classroom in Tibet, I was amazed at how the children could sit silently and motionless for such long stretches of time; I couldn't help imagining how their American equivalents would likely be wiggling their legs and scrolling through the phones they were trying to hide beneath their desks.

But silence is also part of the climate that each therapy session generates. We sense the growing anger of the frustrated mother whose child can't sit still, feel the tension emanating from the struggling couple who sit as far away from each other as possible, or experience the downward pull of sadness from the teen drowning in her grief. Like the weather, the emotional climate is always there in the room, can change in a few moments, and is always part of and envelops the therapeutic chatter.

But while silence is a weather maker, it is different from emotions: We can clearly see the face of some emotions like anger or sadness or anxiety gathering from a distance like a growing storm. Silence, however, can descend suddenly, unexpectedly. And because it can, it can be unnerving, raising your or your client's anxiety. And unlike emotions, it can be a shape-shifter that can take on many faces and forms. Its complexity makes it all the more powerful but also a potential fulcrum for change.

All silences are not created equally. Managing and using silence starts with discerning what type of silence you are dealing with and then knowing how to respond. Here are some common types and their antidotes. We can break them down into those initiated by clients and those created by you.

Client Silences

Angry Silence

Fourteen-year-old Amanda accompanies her parents to their first session. She didn't want to come; she didn't know why she is here, or she thinks "it's their problem," not hers. She's digging in, hunched down in the chair, her arms crossed: "I've got nothing to say," her unique combo of a freeze–fight stress response.

Kudos to Amanda. She picked a pretty good strategy. If therapy is about talking, choosing not to talk is the ultimate process killer—game over. Even if you thought hitting a wall like this might happen, when it does it can raise your anxiety.

Antidote

Say what you think the client is thinking: "I'm guessing that you feel angry that your parents made you come." Or "I realize this must feel awkward." Or "I'm guessing you really don't want to be here." Or "Wow, your parents seem to be giving you a hard time. Do they do that a lot?"

What you're trying to do is get under the client's defenses by empathizing. The key is to sound gentle, be calm, and help her see that you are unlike her parents rather than another scolding adult. Make brief eye contact, and avoid the deep stare. Next say, "I know your parents are worried about some things that you're doing; my job is to help you, and I want to know what you want changed, what you see as the problems that need to be fixed." You've done your best to clarify your role as an advocate for the client rather than as an enforcer for the parents. See if you get a response. If Amanda starts ranting about her parents, let her rant. If you're still getting silence, ask the parents to leave and begin asking off-topic questions—about school, friends, hobbies. Show interest and empathy.

Your goal right now is to get family members to relax and talk, to counter their resistance. The same can happen with a reluctant partner or an elderly parent, who is unsure who you are and why they are there. The content isn't important right now. The focus is on establishing the clinical relationship and creating an environment of safety. Always thank them at the end for talking.

Anxious Silence

But your client may not be angry but anxious. Often clients will freeze up at the start of the initial session even if you've already asked them what they want help with or why they are there. They don't know how to start.

Antidote

Remain silent; avoid eye contact. Your silence will increase their anxiety, and the heightened anxiety will usually push them to start. If it's not working, gently say what you think they're probably thinking: "I realize knowing where to start is hard. Just start anywhere, and I'll help you out."

Overwhelmed Silence

Sam was animated as he talked about his brother but then stopped dead in his tracks. He tilts his head slightly; his eyes suddenly fill with sadness, even tears, or maybe he feels angry in response to your comment. Regardless of the source, the climate in the room has changed; he is emotionally shutting down and is silent.

Antidote

Go quiet. Take a few deep breaths not only to center yourself but because clients will often need to do the same. Gently ask, "What just happened? You look sad (angry)." Your goal is to give them space but to encourage them to put words to their feelings.

Processing Silence

You make an interpretation: "What you've just been saying that bothers you most about your husband sounds a lot like what you said last session about your father and how he treated you when you were a child. I wonder if Jake is triggering some of those old childhood wounds, and that's why you're so upset." Carol goes silent. She is pondering, trying to absorb and process what you said.

Antidote

Give her the time and space she needs. If it is dragging out too long, if you worry that she is perhaps getting lost in her memories, gently pull her back by asking, "Can you tell me what you're thinking?" Again, putting words to an emotional reaction.

Therapist Silences

Overwhelmed Silence

The couple has suddenly turned on you and is blasting you with their frustration. You're stunned and shaken. Eunhee is describing how her older brother sexually abused her as a child, and her story triggers your memories, and your mind starts going down old rabbit holes. You lose track of what she is saying. Unexpectedly, Thom starts talking about his porn addiction, how he obsesses about sex, how he got into trouble on his job last year for watching porn at work, and how he's tried to stop but can't. He turns to you and says, "I'm desperate; I gotta shake this. You gotta help me. What should I do?" You freeze. You have no idea what to say, how to help.

Just as clients can get overwhelmed, so can you by feeling caught off guard, emotionally triggered, or clinically stuck.

Antidote

Take a few deep breaths. Some options: Let them keep talking to give yourself some time to process. If you are getting flooded with too much content—a long story that you're losing track of—shift to emotions in the room: "But I can't tell how you feel about this" or "You're looking sad." If you are getting flooded with too much emotion, shift to content: "Tell me what you've done to try and curb your addiction." "What in particular are you most frustrated by?"

If you don't know why you are overwhelmed, say so: "I'm sorry, I just got mentally distracted. Could you say again what you just said?" "I want to help you with this, but I need to think about what you said and develop a plan that will work best for you. Let me ask you a few more questions, and if you don't mind, I'll have some feedback for you next week."

Silence with Couples and Families

The father is berating his daughter for sneaking out of the house to see her boyfriend. The couple begins to talk about Saturday's argument, but it quickly becomes an emotional brawl with name calling, rising anger, and sarcastic comments.

This is about them, but your silence in such volatile situations is dangerous. It is seen as consent—the teen will not only feel unprotected but think you are siding with her father. The couple will not only realize afterward that they could have done this argument at home for free, but that you are sanctioning how they treat each other and/or that this is what therapy is about.

Antidote

You need to step up and show leadership. Ask the father to calm down; if he can't, hold up your hand and ask him to stop so you can focus on his daughter. Ditto for the couple, and if they can't, then separate them—have one sit in the waiting room while you debrief with the other, and then switch. Don't fail to act.

The many faces of silence. The theme here is decoding what type of silence you're dealing with, seeing it not as a problem but as a form of coping, and using your verbal and nonverbal skills to address the problem beneath the problem.

Can you decode the different faces of silence? Are there certain types that you particularly struggle with? What support do you need; what skills do you need to develop?

CHAPTER 20

Everything to Know about Resistance

Asha seemed motivated for therapy. She said she had been thinking about it for a long time, had done research on different models and clinicians, and for the first few sessions, things were going smoothly: She came with an agenda (learning skills to manage her anxiety), she arrived on time, she did the homework you suggested, she even recommended you to one of her friends. But then something shifted. Asha missed a couple of appointments in a row, citing "work issues"; she wasn't doing the homework; she seemed distracted or scattered during sessions. What's going on?

Ah, the face of resistance. Now, if you are steeped in psychodynamic therapy, you probably aren't surprised—you knew this would eventually happen. It's baked into the process. Clients want to change but resist change: the yin and yang, the tug of war. But it doesn't need to be that inevitable or complicated. Here is my list of the four common sources of client resistance and their antidotes.

1. No Agreement about the Problem

"So, I don't think we need to be here."

"Okay. Can you tell me why?"

"You see, the problem is that I can't mix vodka and beer."

Jake is all elbows and angles, while his wife Maggie is round and doughy. According to the intake sheet, the court ordered Jake and his wife Maggie to go to couples counseling. During a particularly loud argument, neighbors called the police, who came to the home and ultimately decided to charge each of them with assault. The judge in the case ordered them to come to see you.

"I don't understand."

"Well," says Jake, punctuating the air for emphasis, "I learned a long time ago that I can't mix beer and vodka; I just get crazy, so I've stayed a beer drinker. But my oldest son came over a few weeks ago and brought a bottle of vodka that a friend had given him who said this was the best vodka since the beginning of time. So I tried it, I was curious, but I should've known better. But then I got crazy, and Maggie and I got into it—I really didn't mean to hit you, honey," he says, turning toward her. "But I've learned my lesson; I'm off the vodka and sticking to beer. And we've been doing good since then, haven't we, honey?"

Maggie pipes up: "Yeah, we've been doing good."

"So," says Jake, "we don't really need to be here."

I actually had this exchange with a couple many years ago and, maybe like you, I was a bit stuck about what to say next. The therapeutic process just came to a halt because Jake and Maggie felt there was no problem, or maybe there was a problem, but in their minds, an isolated event that has been since taken care of. Since there's nothing to fix, there's no need to be there.

Antidote

Jake and Maggie are clearly not seeing the problem in the same way the community is. They see what happened as a one-time vodka-driven event, while the community is concerned about potentially ongoing domestic violence. What you want to do in these situations, especially when a court order is hanging over their heads and yours (the court or social services expects you to provide reports about attendance and progress), is to start by clarifying who has the problem and who is the customer.

To avoid getting lost in the weeds of whose reality is right, invite the community members to the first session: Call in the probation officer or someone from the prosecutor's office to air their concerns. Instead of being seen as the cop, you can let the complainants speak for themselves. With their concerns on the table, you now have solid facts and words that you can weave into your future sessions with the client: Mr. Jones didn't say that the vodka wasn't a factor; what I heard him say is that domestic violence is rarely an isolated event or stays an isolated event and that he wanted you to get the help that you might need. If you can't get the community rep to talk to you for whatever reason, make sure you do have accurate information, such as a copy of the court order.

If Jake and Maggie are not buying into the community's view of the problem, your Plan B is to find another problem that does: The only thing that usually motivates people are problems—theirs, not someone else's. Jake and Maggie may be willing to see you simply to get the court or social services off their backs. Or you may say to Jake and Maggie that you understand how they feel that the court is maybe making a big deal about nothing. Still, you're wondering how to help the couple handle differences even in better times or how their children may feel after witnessing their altercation.

This plan can obviously be a hard sell, especially if they are suspicious of outside agencies and help, but you present it in hopes of finding common ground you all can build around. It's not about moving toward the right change but bringing the notion of change into the relationship and larger system.

2. No Agreement about the Solution

Or the resistance isn't about the problem but about the solution, namely therapy. Jake and Maggie agree that maybe their relationship could use some help, but they don't want to talk to you because they're not crazy or because you're a stranger and they don't need to talk with a stranger about something that is clearly none of your business.

Or the resistance isn't about therapy itself, but about the solutions you are proposing. By the second session, you're terribly concerned that Jake has a serious alcohol problem or that he is massively depressed, possibly driving the drinking. You express your concerns and suggest that he consider a consultation with a colleague who specializes in substance issues or that he talk with his family doctor about possible medication. But he says he doesn't have a problem with alcohol, so he doesn't want to speak to a specialist; he's against medication and isn't willing to consider it, so he doesn't need to see his doctor.

Antidote

The problem is the problem in the room, namely, that you're on different pages. You want to focus on deconstructing the resistance: "I understand that talking to a stranger seems weird. This is not about your being crazy—you're not—but simply being an outsider who isn't biased may help me help you figure out possible ways to solve your problem. Are you willing to try it for a couple of sessions?" Or, to a client who is resisting your suggestion to consider medication: "You say you don't believe in medication. Can you tell me why? What bothers you about it?" Or "I'm suggesting talking to your doctor because ____________. Does this make sense?" You're dealing with resistance by attempting to deconstruct it.

3. Different Expectations about the Process

Jake and Maggie expected to come in once, that you would chat with them for the session, then write a letter to the court to say that they came. Asha thought you would move through a list of anxiety-managing skills, but when you become concerned that much of her anxiety may stem from past childhood trauma and ask questions about her childhood experiences, she gets skittish, anxious, and drops out. Or the problem is around administrative expectations: Your agency has a ten-session or three-month cap on treatment, but Charles wasn't told about the policy and was expecting ongoing longer-term treatment.

Finally, the problem may be about the pace of the process. You suggest that Asha experiment with mindfulness meditation to help her settle when her anxiety begins to ramp up. You explained the technique to her; she says she understands it, but then she doesn't do it; she says it was a busy week and she didn't have time to try it. You can see this response as resistance, but it may be about your pacing. Asha said she understood what to do, but maybe she didn't. Or she doesn't understand how meditation will help her in the present when she is overwhelmed. Or she asked about techniques, but you are offering too many at once and she can't process them all. The pace is too fast.

But for other clients, your pacing may be too slow. Sixteen-year-old Tesha's parents drag her into an initial session because they just learned she is cutting. You listen to their and Tesha's concerns. At the end of the session, and with Tesha's agreement, you say to the parents that you want to do three individual sessions with her for further evaluation, and then you would all meet again as a family to decide on the next steps. But this is not at all what the parents were expecting. They thought you would do a white-coat intervention, pull Tesha aside, and say some magic words that would "straighten her out," or that you would at least provide some immediate feedback right away.

Antidote

Be clear about your model and style at the front end and clarify any administrative policies and concerns. When there seems to be agreement but lack of follow-through—homework isn't being done, clients cancel the next appointment—something was amiss. Proactively you want to make sure there is a solid commitment to following your suggestions and a preliminary plan during the session. Look for any signs of confusion or resistance as the process unfolds, especially in those crucial opening sessions.

4. Transference Issues

This problem is trickier. There is positive transference, where you remind your client of her brother, whom she adores with his laid-back attitude and sense of humor. Or a negative transference, where you remind her of her brother, who is always critical and competitive. The negative one can block rapport and trigger emotional reactions that keep clients from hearing or accepting anything you say. Basically, from their perspective, they walk out feeling that they just don't like you; it's not a good fit. But it's not about you.

One of your major challenges in working with clients is doing your best not to trigger these negative transferences to avoid creating resistance. Here we can imagine that Jake and Maggie are in part resistant because the community is stepping in and telling them what to do; they feel intruded upon and micromanaged. Knowing that they are sensitive to community judgment and control, you need to be careful about your own approach within a session to not replicate the problem—by sounding aggressive or demanding or by minimizing their point of view. You want to watch your tone so that you don't sound too harsh; you reassure them yet again that you understand what they are saying and are wanting to better understand the problem. And if you still encounter resistance, you can move to Plan B: Return to their motivating problem—finding ways to get the community to leave them alone. Be their ally rather than another source of conflict.

This is about shaping the therapy, not to make it your therapy, but to actively work around clients' transferences that can get in the way of building a therapeutic relationship. Crafting the therapeutic relationship is your responsibility. If you go on autopilot—you doing you, responding essentially the same way with everyone—your clients will do the same—doing what they do, seeing you through the same, well-worn lens; you end up with a stalemate. And making this challenge even more challenging, you ideally need to identify these negative transferences as quickly as possible.

Antidote

One easy way of identifying transference is what we previously discussed, listening for *transference cues*. As clients talk about their current and past relationships, you have a wealth of important information: Your client talks about the way her father was critical, or her partner is silent and shuts down, or her best friend always interrupts and pushes her advice on the client. In a few sentences, you learned a great deal: that the client is sensitive to criticism and to passivity and not feeling engaged and that interruptions and too-ready advice push her buttons. You now know what not to do to avoid triggering her old wounds and seeing you as "one of them." This does not mean you have to walk on eggshells and duct-tape your mouth shut. It means that you need to be more sensitive to not triggering the client.

So if Asha is sensitive to criticism, you say before making a suggestion or asking a hard question, "I'm not trying to sound critical, but I'm wondering about . . . " For the client complaining about her passive partner, you deliberately step up and ask a question as she goes on and on in a story about her past. Or, for the client who feels interrupted, you try to be the ideal listener and give her space to speak. You are not walking on eggshells, not letting her run the therapy, nor being passive, but are sensitive to what these clients need that they never received. You are proactively shaping the conversation to minimize emotional resistance so that they can hear you better when you explain your perspective, your concerns, your reframing of their problem, and your treatment plan. You are offering them a new vision of the problem and the path to success so that they can best absorb what you are saying. You are deciding how to be that ideal parent or partner so you have a better way of entering their lives.

The theme that runs through all of these sources of resistance is that they are less about the client and more about you. Yes, resistance may and likely will arise, but you can both anticipate and manage it. By doing this, you're doing the best you can do.

As with other skill sets, this is another one to explore and experiment with and, like others, you can start outside the office. To be more sensitive to transference cues, try listening to friends or to your family's stories about others and pay attention to how they describe others from their past and present; decode what they are most sensitive to. Listen for when your suggestions to a friend seem dismissed, when your partner seems less than excited about your plans for his birthday. The goal here is to become sensitive to when resistance is unfolding, when the conversation has been blocked, and when what you say isn't having the effect you hoped.

CHAPTER 21

Getting on Track and Staying There

You're looking at the day's new intake forms: A woman is struggling with depression, a couple with "communication problems"; a family with a teen "who has an attitude." You feel that flutter of anxiety. You're not feeling all that concerned about the woman with depression, but you find yourself wondering if the couple is way older than you or whether they are going to be arguing in the session; you don't know what "an attitude" means, but you already know the teen is not going to be happy to be there. And, it being the first session, you're aware that you've got a lot to cover—paperwork, building some rapport, defining goals, starting an assessment, and even hopefully offering a preliminary treatment plan—all the awkwardness of a first date with the added performance pressure of earning your keep.

You're right to feel anxious—even the most seasoned clinicians can get that flutter. And you're right about the pressure. If what you're thinking isn't enough to cause you to hyperventilate, we can always throw on top of your anxiety pile the fact that most folks only go to therapy once (Brown et al., 2005). What this means is that if you want them to return, you need to help them feel better when they walk out than when they walked in. Did anyone mention pressure?

It may be helpful to talk with experienced colleagues to see how they've developed their style and format to navigate their first sessions. But if you're looking for a universal model to give you some grounding, there's probably no better place to start than looking at how family doctors handle their appointments. Like you, they too are seeing a variety of patients with various presenting problems, and they too want them to feel better when they walk out than when they walked in. But adding to their challenge is that they generally only have fifteen to twenty minutes to do their magic, while you have the luxury of seeing clients for 50 minutes or an hour. So take a moment and think about your last couple of doctor appointments.

You have this rash on your arm. You have no idea where it came from, but you're freaking out—it burns, it itches, and it looks like it's spreading. You go on WebMD and look it up, and that freaks you out even more—photos of things like African mange or some skin-rotting disease show up. Now your anxiety is going through the roof. You call your doctor; she can see you at 2:00. Whew.

You show up. She asks why you are there. You show her your arm; tell her you're worried; you mention the African mange that you think looks just like your rash. She listens carefully and looks at it more closely—with a magnifying glass, strong lights. Then she asks you questions: How long have you had this? Does it itch or burn? All the time, some of the time? Do you have allergies? Have you been out in the woods? What have you done to manage it—ice, heat, or creams? Did they help?

And then she gives you her diagnosis: "I think you have contact dermatitis. Don't worry; it's not African mange, because African mange really only happens in Africa. You said that you were out in the woods, and it's easy to rub against some poisonous plant without even realizing it, and your symptoms match those of contact dermatitis. Here is a prescription; actually, here is a free sample for a cream to apply. Use it for three days. If it is not better, seems to be getting worse, let me know, and I will order some labwork just to see if something more systemic is going on."

Do you feel better when you walk out than when you walked in? Absolutely. And you're out the door in fifteen minutes.

So what just happened? What did she do that worked? Let's break it down.

Have Treatment Maps

She is not a dermatologist, but as a primary care physician, she probably has in her repertoire a dozen common skin conditions that she regularly sees and knows how to treat. If you said you had just returned from Africa and showed up with something she didn't recognize, she would probably refer you to a dermatologist. But the conditions she knows, she knows. She's seen enough contact dermatitis to identify it, and she reduces her usual suspects to a few with her questions. And once she's settled on one, she knows about two or three remedies that will probably work.

She can hit the ground running because she has treatment maps in her head about treating common skin conditions; she already has several possible hypotheses ready to go. She doesn't have to run off to her office, look up journal articles on her computer, or take blood samples for everyone she sees. Instead, she listens, looks, narrows down the possibilities, then can quickly plug in her version of the treatment plan—the cream for three days.

You want to do the same—have in your clinical bag of tricks maps of common problems you're most likely to see already on board: generalized anxiety, children with ADHD, situational depression, parents who are polarized around parenting—whatever is common to your client population and job. With these maps, you, like your doctor, avoid having to invent the wheel for every session; by having them mentally in place, you quickly narrow down the problem and what you are looking for; and once it is at least preliminarily confirmed, you are ready to offer a preliminary treatment plan. By having this plan in place ahead of time, your anxiety decreases. You feel mentally prepared and in control.

Track the Process like a Bloodhound

Your doctor mentions that if the creams don't seem to work, there are some oral medications that you can take, and you tell her that you can't swallow pills. Similarly, you may say to your client struggling with depression, "I wonder if what you're describing as depression is actually grief tied to the recent loss of your father," and your client makes a face and slightly shakes her head. You and your doctor have a problem in the room; her patient and your client are out of step with her and with you.

To ensure that your client will be on board when you present your preliminary treatment plan and feel better when he walks out than when he walked in, you, like your doctor, need to make sure that you and your client stay in lockstep as you move through the session. At any point in the process when you make an interpretation, prescribe homework, talk about next steps, or provide information, you want to listen carefully to what the client does next. You're looking for solid agreement by a nod of the head, by a verbal "Yes, that makes sense."

If you don't, but instead get a confused look or a half-hearted okay, you need to stop and address the problem: "I noticed you are shaking your head. It seems like you might be thinking about this differently; tell me how you are thinking about this." Or "You look confused. The reason I was saying this is because ____________." If you ignore these negative reactions, the client may balk at your treatment plan, not do the homework, or simply not return. You want to track the process like a bloodhound; make sure that you and the client are in lockstep, that there is consensus throughout the session.

Control the Clock

A well-known dictum in football is: He who controls the clock controls the game—deciding to run out the clock versus throwing passes to save time; calling time-outs to slow the momentum of the other team, or coming up with the best plan to use the time that is left. With your limited time and your own goals, you're in a similar position; you too want to control the clock. If you don't, you won't finish your assessment and can only punt at the end of the session, saying we'll need to continue this conversation next time. If you don't, the husband will rant about his partner for 40 minutes, leaving you with no time to hear the spouse's side of the story or even wrap up. The partner will leave feeling dismissed—yet again—and you'll probably feel the same, a bit shell-shocked.

Controlling the clock involves two steps. The first is keeping an eye on how time is passing and how much time you have left in your session—be aware of time itself as another part of the unfolding therapy process. The second is about control: Planning how you want to use the time in the session and then managing how the process unfolds. I tend to think of the first session in three parts, and I think your family doctor is likely doing the same.

Part One is the opening. Here your doctor asks what brings you in, and you talk about the rash on your arm. Your equivalent is helping the client get settled, build some rapport, find out why she is there—that she is waking up and obsessing in the middle of the night, or that the couple is arguing all the time, or that the teen says "no" to everything—the presenting problem. Part Two is your assessment: Your doctor starts asking questions to sort through and confirm her hypothesis. Here you do the same based on your clinical model—ask about symptoms, past history, drill down on thoughts and behaviors—whatever information you need to confirm your diagnosis.

In Part Three, present your diagnosis and a preliminary treatment plan. The doctor says it's contact dermatitis; here is a cream to use. You say it's understandable that you feel depressed because of your recent loss, that the couple's understandably triggering each other and struggling to regulate their emotions, that the teen says she feels like her parents are micromanaging, treating her like a six-year-old rather than the sixteen-year-old that she is. You say that to help you with your grief, you need to get closure—here is an exercise you can do. You lay out a behavior plan to help the couple realize when their emotions are getting out of control. You tell the family that you'd like each of them to come up with a list of topics that bother them most and that in the next session, you will help them negotiate a plan that works for all of them.

But the clock is ticking, and you need to watch it. Give each part fifteen minutes. Setting a time limit will help you keep the husband from ranting or the individual client from going on and on about her past with little time to mop up.

So there you have it, the triad—treatment maps, tracking the process like a bloodhound, and controlling the clock; together, they provide a solid foundation for managing those anxiety-producing first sessions.

Think about your own experiences with first sessions. Are there treatment maps missing from your clinical inventory that you need to develop? Do you need to pay more attention to the clock and pacing? Can you notice when a client is out of step with you? Talk these issues over with your supervisor, perhaps sit in on one of your seasoned colleagues' first sessions, or watch training videos to see how others manage these challenges. As you gain experience, you'll undoubtedly find ways to integrate these skills into your particular style and personality.

CHAPTER 22

Changing the Emotional Climate

No doubt you have specific goals for your client sessions. If it's the first session, you want to know the presenting problems, to define symptoms, to likely gather family history, and to track past treatment in order to come up with a preliminary diagnosis. If it's a later session, you may want to discuss setting up a team meeting with the client's other providers or repairing your relationship with the husband, who you worry may have felt criticized and ganged up on in the session before. What you decide to put on your agenda will obviously vary based on your and the client's evolving needs. But there's another agenda item that you want to make sure you consider—shaping and changing the emotional climate.

As the term implies, the emotional climate is like the weather, ever-present and often quickly changeable. Sometimes the change is precipitated by content—high-fives when your client who has been struggling with anorexia proudly announces that she put on three pounds in the past week—but it is quickly nullified by her news that her grandmother is terminally ill with cancer. At other times, it's the climate driving the content—your client's overwhelming sadness leads her to spend the session recalling memories of her time with her grandmother and her imagined life without her. Here the climate naturally changes as the session unfolds.

But sometimes you want to be more intentional, not just noticing what evolves but proactively shaping the process to shift the session's tone, repair a relationship, or ensure that the clients leave feeling differently when they leave compared to when they came in. How do you do this?

Here are some techniques to consider and experiment with.

Focus on the Underlying Soft or Hard Emotions

Tim angrily complains to his teenage daughter, Sam, about how she rolls her eyes and does this shrug anytime he offers her advice about managing her time better. On and on he goes; he's frustrated and feels dismissed. "But what are you most worried about?" you ask Tim gently. His face slackens. "That she'll wind up struggling like I did when I was her age. That she too will wind up feeling like a failure."

Tolu's supervisor has called her on the carpet again about coming to work late. "It's my fault," she says in her mumbled, depressed, self-critical way. "Sure," you say. "I understand that it is ultimately your responsibility to get to work on time. But I also remember you telling me several times that many folks on your team are also late, and your supervisor never says anything about their behavior to them. I think if I always felt singled out, picked on, and treated differently from everyone else, I would feel that it was unfair. I could imagine feeling deep down frustrated, angry even. Do you ever feel that way?"

A powerful way of changing the climate is focusing on the "opposite" underlying emotions that are not expressed or said. Sam is familiar with Tim's default go-to anger that fills the space at home and in the session, triggering Sam's tuned-out, dismissive reaction. And so, we ask about what Tim is not saying or expressing—the anxiety driving his micromanaging—and deliberately speak softly to get under his defenses. With the shift in emotion, Sam can hear and see her father in a new way.

For Tolu, we're moving in the other direction. In contrast to Tim, her default is internalization, self-criticism, that classic "depression as anger turned inward." By using a stronger voice, by saying how we might feel, we are actively changing the tone in the room, modeling and hopefully encouraging her to expand her emotional range, look deeper into her response, and verbalize how she may feel and think differently.

By going where the clients are not, tapping into those opposite emotions, the climate is quickly changed, and with it often comes a shift in the conversation and perspective.

Tap into Nonverbal Cues

In a similar vein, you can focus on unacknowledged nonverbal cues. Tim does his rant, but you notice that his eyes look teary; Tolu mumbles "my fault," but you see that her fists are clenched as she says this. Rather than tracking the words, you focus on these physical reactions: "Tim, you sound angry, but your eyes look sad; what's going on?" again in a gentle voice. "Tolu, you're blaming yourself, but I notice that your hands are clenched. What might your hands be saying if they could talk?"

Demonstrate the Ideal Voice

You see Tim without Sam, and he again sounds angry and frustrated. You say to him, "I'm wondering what would happen if after a confrontation, after you've cooled down, you gently said to Sam, 'I'm sorry I gave you a hard time yesterday about managing your time. I know I sounded angry and frustrated, but I'm worried. You seem to be always struggling with your schoolwork; I know you feel that I'm on your back. But I'm afraid that you will get discouraged or give up or begin to feel like a failure if you can't keep up. I love you and don't want it to happen.' What do you think your daughter would say if you said that?"

What you might expect is that Tim would soften. But more important, by your verbalizing what he ideally could say, you are tapping into his underlying emotions, role modeling for him a different way of communicating with his daughter and offering a way of changing the dynamics of the relationship. If you saw Sam by herself and said the same to her—"Suppose your father said . . ."—she too would possibly see her father's behavior in a new light. Similarly, you could verbalize for Tolu how she might assertively talk with her supervisor about her feeling singled out.

Think of the ideal voice as a one-sided role play where you express what is not said but likely needs to be said more clearly. It's less about conveying facts and more about modeling how to express emotions differently and more effectively, in a more assertive, honest, and often compassionate way.

Stage an Enactment

You ask Tim and Sam to discuss in the session how to work together and develop a win–win plan that helps reduce Tim's worry and keeps

Sam from feeling micromanaged. Here you are the sideline coach, steering the conversation to focus on those softer emotions and allow each of them to feel heard while keeping the conversation moving toward a resolution.

Reframe the Problem

Tim and Sam have stopped their battles, but Tim still feels that Sam is simply not trying hard enough, not making her schoolwork a priority. You say, "Tim, I remember you mentioning a few weeks ago that you too struggled in school and that looking back on it, your dad was always procrastinating and forgetful, and your mom was constantly aggravated by his not following through on things. I'm wondering aloud whether all three of you have an attention disorder. It is genetic and runs in families. When it's not diagnosed and left untreated, it can cause the problems you've described—difficulty focusing, completing tasks, setting priorities, meeting deadlines. I'm wondering if it might be something that you and Sam might want to have evaluated. How does that sound?"

We could do something similar with Tolu: "It does seem like your supervisor is treating you unfairly, and it probably would be good if we could come up with a better way of talking with her about how you have been feeling. I know you are reluctant to do this and feel intimidated by her. But I'm also concerned about how easily you blame yourself for this and many things in your life. You initially came for depression, and often folks prone to depression tend to hold things in and get angry with themselves rather than with others. While this problem is about your work and your supervisor, I think this is also a challenge and opportunity for you—to not be so self-critical and to be kinder to yourself, to learn to push back against your fears. Does this make sense? Is this something you are willing to work on?"

We're certainly talking here about diagnoses, but the process is about reframing—essentially giving clients new problems to replace the worn-out ones they struggle to solve. With a new perspective and a new challenge, they leave the session with a new frame of reference and a new goal, which give them new energy and motivation.

Educate

You give Tim and Sam some handouts on attention-deficit disorders; you describe to Tolu the characteristics of depression and the personality of people prone to it. While reframing helps clients see their problems in a different light, educating them about the symptoms and etiology of their problems, about the overall patterns of their relationship, about the influence of history and genetics, or about the way their brains respond to their stress provides a broader and often normalizing context. The client leaves feeling more grounded, more enlightened, and less anxious.

Offer a Clear Treatment Plan

This is about creating hope, a light at the end of the tunnel. This is where you refer Tim and Sam to a physician specializing in ADHD or a psychologist who can do testing. This is where you say to Tolu that next time you could role-play talking with her supervisor or talk about some techniques that she can try to tackle her self-criticism.

The themes here are several. One is that proactively changing the emotional climate is something that you may want to consider at the top of a session—the "How do I ideally want the client to feel differently when he walks out than when he walked in?" It is also about learning the tricky skill of paying attention to content while tracking the emotional climate—like moving between process and content. It is about having tools and techniques at the ready so you can shape the climate as it unfolds when you need it to.

Yes, all these techniques may seem challenging to learn and master. Again, pick one or two to focus on. Practice applying them not only with clients, but even with friends and family outside of work. Experiment, for example, using the ideal voice with a friend who is angry at his parent, or when you're out to lunch with your partner or friend, simply paying attention to and picking up on nonverbal cues. Like other skill sets, it is not about personality but about practice. It will get easier over time and, as always, it's okay to make mistakes.

CHAPTER 23

The Challenge of Couple Therapy

Anya and Kamil are sitting across from you. It's their first session, not only with you, but also with couple therapy. Anya has had individual therapy in the past; Kamil has not. You do your preliminary tasks—signing forms and introducing them to you and the agency. But then, as you do with every new client, you turn the corner and say, "How can I help? What brings you here today?"

And all hell breaks loose. Anya is up and running: "The reason why we're here is that we can't communicate; we get into stupid arguments; he's always hitting me up for sex at 11:00 at night after I've been up with the kids since 6:00 A.M.; he hates my mother; he forgot our anniversary; he drinks too much!"

You turn to Kamil: "What do you think about what Anya is saying? What are you worried about?"

You might get a shrug and an "I don't know; this was her idea," before he slumps into passivity. Or, he's up with his own counterattack: "I try to talk with her, but she goes ballistic in five seconds; we get into stupid arguments because she is so critical and picky about everything; I don't hit her up for sex but *suggest* it, and she's always not in the mood; I don't hate her mother, but her mother can be a pain, and I've said that to her but she doesn't do anything about it; I admit I did forget our anniversary, but she got me an Amazon gift card for my birthday—last minute, I think; I don't drink too much, I only have a couple of beers after a hard day at work, but because her dad was an alcoholic, she thinks everyone is . . . "

Welcome to the world of couple therapy.

I think that couple therapy is one of the most challenging forms of therapy to navigate. Unlike individual therapy, you lose the intimacy it naturally creates—the one-on-one, the uninterrupted give and take. You can more easily track the narrative and clients' emotions as they naturally unfold in the session—and how do they make you feel? And if a client tears up or cries or is openly angry, it's easy to be empathic; or if you are getting lost in the story, you can back it up to gain clarity because you have a singular focus.

And unlike family therapy, couple therapy lacks the built-in family's cotherapists who can ask the hard questions. "But why are you always angry with me?" asks the eight-year-old or the teen who reveals family secrets: "But you smoke pot too, Dad." In family therapy, you become more the traffic cop who is holding up your hand and trying to manage or redirect the conversational traffic: "Hold on, Jim. Let Ann speak"; "Wait a minute, Tom. You sound like you're scolding Billy; tell him what you're most worried about." You guide and shape the unfolding process to move it in a positive direction. But couple therapy lacks that intimacy and natural momentum. It can feel more like a cockfight, a courtroom scene with opposing sides, a traffic jam with each partner unwilling to yield any right of way.

If you're feeling a bit discouraged at the notion of taking this all on, that's understandable. Here are some suggestions to help you handle these challenges.

Demonstrate Leadership

If you let Anya and Kamil do what they do, they will not only think that therapy is a waste of time because they essentially did what they could have done at home for free, but they will also walk away feeling that you couldn't provide what they needed most—a person and a place to feel safe. There's a good chance they won't be back. The safety they need comes from your strong leadership, from exercising some control, and from stepping up even though it's easy to feel overwhelmed, and you want to duck for cover in the face of all that is coming at you. To act in spite of how you might feel, you need to be mentally prepared, pumped up as you might be before an athletic competition or a stage performance. You want to adopt a take-charge attitude before they walk in the front door.

Create Balance

Your leadership sets a tone of safety by essentially conveying the message to each partner: "I've got your back." But to make them each believe that, you need to make sure that you've got each of their backs equally. This is about creating a balance that is so crucial to couple therapy. Unlike individual or family therapy, where you're dealing with one-on-one or one-on-many, couple therapy is naturally unbalanced simply because of the triangle in the room—it's always two against one—you and Anya, you and Kamil, Anya and Kamil versus you. Just as you can't afford to have Anya and Kamil do what they already can do in their own home, you also can't afford for one of them to walk out feeling as though you were biased and felt left out.

The skill set here is always keeping the need for balance in mind and then detecting any subtle shifts in the balance as it unfolds. You don't want Anya, for example, to dominate the session with a rant or break down and cry, nor do you want Kamil to do the same. If you sense that Anya felt interrupted or cut off, explain why you did what you did. You need to watch the clock and control the process—by deliberately not asking deeper questions about one partner's anger if you know you don't have time to focus on the other. Keep your session goals in mind.

And if your style is to see the individuals separately first, make sure you see both of them before seeing them together; if one partner cannot make an appointment for whatever reason, balance it out by offering an individual appointment before seeing them again as a couple to counter their paranoia and often their expectation that you are biased.

Don't Play Courtroom

If the inherent triangle of couple work isn't enough to manage, their differing realities often add to the fire, even in couples who have been in therapy before. Often their individual goals are to present the *true facts* and have you agree that their versions of the truth are correct: "Yes, Anya is clearly overly emotional"; "Yes, Kamil has a drinking problem." Don't do this. They are using therapy as a courtroom, seeing you as the judge, but therapy is not a courtroom. Instead, step up and call them on their expectations and the tit-for-tat process. Let them know at the start and in midsession that your job is not to play judge and decide whose reality is right but to help them learn to solve their problems. That said, they will test—"But you heard what he just said: Am I the crazy one here?" Take a deep breath and restate your position.

Control the Emotions

Because safety is created not by wading through the facts and deciding whose story makes sense, you want to focus on controlling the emotional temperature and climate in the room. If Anya or Kamil ramps up, your goal is to lower the temperature. Here you can say, "Kamil, you seem to be getting angry. Can you tell you're getting upset because of what Anya said?"; "I understand you both are feeling upset. I'm not being critical, but I'd like to lower the emotional temperature in the room. Can you both try and take a couple of deep breaths to help yourselves settle a bit?"

By speaking in this way, you are doing a few things: showing leadership and stopping them from replicating the problem in the room, demonstrating how to change the climate by being aware of the process, and then teaching them new skills. Once they have settled, you can explain to them what you just did and why—that you weren't trying to cut them off, or being critical, but that you are trying to help them become more sensitive to when their emotions take over the conversation and to what leads to their arguments. Undoubtedly, you will have to control the emotional climate many times: Kamil or Anya may continue to ramp up, but you hold steady and repeat your suggestion calmly.

And what if you can't rein in Kamil or Anya? Separate them. Don't try to slog through a session feeling overwhelmed by all the he-said, she-said; they will wind up feeling frustrated. Again, take control, be a leader. Ask Anya to sit in the waiting room while you talk to Kamil for a few minutes. But be aware of the clock and the need for balance. If you run out of time and don't circle back to Anya, she'll walk away thinking, "Yes, Kamil obviously is the problem; I was right," or you heard his view of the problem and are now on his side. Instead, settle Kamil, but then have Anya return and express her side of the problem or see her individually at the start of the next session.

Watch the Clock

Enough said. Don't be afraid to step and shift gears: "I realize that we only have fifteen minutes left. Before we end, there are some questions I need to ask; I want to hear what Kamil is thinking."

Be Aware of Your Countertransference

It's all too easy for couple therapy to hit home on many levels. If you are struggling in your personal relationship, you may too easily identify with Anya's or with Kamil's arguments. If they remind you of your parents, not only might you identify with them, but you too easily can fall into the "little-kid" role, in which you feel small and powerless and revert to your past coping patterns of withdrawing, accommodating, or getting angry.

The key here is knowing yourself and your vulnerabilities at the start. If you see on the intake sheet that the husband is ex-military and is 30 years older than you—all a bit too close to home—consider your possible triggers in advance and map out what you need to do to counter them. Similarly, if you're struggling in your personal relationship and are even thinking of divorce, you need to go into the sessions knowing that you are in danger of projecting your challenges onto them, vicariously having them fight out your battles, or even pushing them toward the divorce you're afraid to get.

As always, here you need an awareness of yourself and get support and a reality check with your supervisor or a trusted colleague.

Mop Up

And if a session becomes unbalanced despite your efforts, you want to mop up. You may want to wait until the next session and start with that—saying to Anya, for example, that you realize that you ran out of time and didn't give her enough chance to share her concerns. If you are afraid that Anya left in a huff and felt dismissed, email, text, or call her, saying that you're sorry that you ran over and she didn't get to tell her side of the story. What you're conveying is your awareness of what unfolded and your concern that both partners feel heard. Again, it's not about balancing content but balancing out the imbalance.

Again, as we said at the beginning, couple therapy is tough because of its unique challenges. If you can learn to avoid these common pitfalls, you'll do fine.

CHAPTER 24

Three Big Obstacles in Relationships

To manage all the information and emotion that emerge with seeing couples and families, it helps to supplement your foundational clinical model with a conceptual framework that can guide you through the relationship maze. Here's one for you to consider and experiment with. It can help you move through that critical first session and provide you with a quick assessment that you can share with the couple or family.

1. Communication

You have heard a thousand times about the importance of good communication, and undoubtedly so have your clients. Yet often they don't communicate, so stuff builds up. One gets too angry too quickly, and the other guy shuts down. Or they slide again into Christmas 2018, or *that* comment someone made to the other's mother as they went out the door two years ago, and everything turns explosive and hurtful.

The good news about communication is that it's a skill that clients can learn and, like any skill, it gets better with concentration and practice. The bad news is that it can be hard to help clients learn to communicate, simply because couples and families have a history: they know how to push each other's emotional buttons. To introduce communication skills to clients, here is how I explain the skills to couples:

Having a conversation is like driving a car. There are two parts to driving a car. Before getting in the car, you need to decide where you want to go. If the conversation has a purpose—deciding on the kids' bedtime, fine-tuning the budget, sorting out what happened on Tuesday—be clear about the point of the discussion, where you want to go, before you start.

The other part of driving is keeping the car on the road, and this is where most couples and families get stuck. When people become emotional, their amygdalas—the emotional center of the brain—fire up and knock their rational brains off-line. They get tunnel vision and want to get others to understand what they're saying; they start stacking up evidence to make their case—going back to Christmas 2018, pulling out texts, repeating what the mother said. And once the conversation heats up, the topic they intended to talk about is no longer on the table; the topic now is the emotions themselves, and anything they say at this point is like throwing gasoline on a fire.

Your first line of defense in these situations is to be quiet and talk about feelings—"You seem to be getting upset. I'm not trying to give you a hard time. What's wrong?" The key is to say these words calmly and to listen and allow the other person to talk. The skill is learning to fix feelings with feelings, not with facts, and lower the emotional temperature.

But if you both are getting upset, the car is off the road and is getting stuck in the mud. It's time to stop the car. Here you need to say, "I'm getting upset" (not, "You're getting upset") "and I need to take a break to calm down. I'll come back in an hour." Knowing that you're coming back helps the other party from feeling cut off and frustrated that the upsetting issue will not be resolved.

Skilled communication when faced with a sensitive topic requires emotional regulation and taking responsibility. It requires each party talking about themselves: their feelings, their intentions, their worries. It's important to avoid talking about the other guy, to resist arguing over whose reality is right, and most of all, to control your temper and keep the conversation moving forward toward some solution. (We're back to our concept of being adult; see Chapter 8.)

Finally, the couple (or family) needs to get the car back on the road once the dust has settled. It is not about simply making up—I'm sorry; are we okay?—but circling back and having a sane two-part conversation. Part A is returning to the topic and formulating a plan to solve the problem. Part B is talking about communication itself—the story of the argument and the lesson learned: Why did they each get upset?

"Because you were interrupting and not listening"; "Because I felt you were talking down to me, scolding me as though I am a child." It's good to know where and how an earlier conversation went haywire.

What to Do

You want to track this process as it unfolds. Are they getting defensive, arguing over facts; can they rein it in? If the conversation heats up, give them a few beats to see if they can self-regulate. If not, you want to stop them; the car is going off the road. You point this out, get them back on track. Ask about circling back and solving problems—can they do this? If not, why not?

2. Childhood Wounds

The notion of childhood wounds goes like this: We all emerge from our childhoods sensitive to a handful of things—feeling criticized, micromanaged, not appreciated, neglected, or dismissed—all based on how our parents treated us. As a child, we only have three ways to cope with the world: withdrawal, being good and walking on eggshells, or getting angry. And if we have siblings, we often navigate by seeing ourselves in comparison to them—my brother is the quiet one, my sister, the angry one, I'm the good one. This works in that it helps us cope when we feel or anticipate feeling wounded.

At some point in a relationship, our partner, a parent, or a child inadvertently triggers these wounds—complains about the way you painted the wall and you feel criticized; suggests how to get to Walmart and you feel micromanaged; doesn't comment on the lovely dinner you spent hours making and you feel unappreciated; doesn't respond to your text for six hours and you feel neglected; interrupts you when you are talking about your day or blows off your suggestion for a vacation and you feel dismissed. When this happens, you immediately do what you learned to do—withdraw, accommodate, or get annoyed. Frequently, as soon as you respond in one of these ways, your response sets off the other's wounds and coping style: The person feels, say, dismissed and gets angry, you withdraw, the other feels even more dismissed, you withdraw further, or you both get mad; everybody is feeling wounded, each is fueling the other and the argument, creating a negative loop. Around and around this goes until one of you storms out or acts out, breaking the cycle for now. But if the cycle continues, eventually someone is going to get fed up: "I'm sick and tired of feeling ____________" (fill in the blank). The couple decides to separate; the family members lapse into a cold war.

The way out of the process is breaking the loop, getting the partners or family members to help heal each other's wounds, rather than continuing to rewound each other. How to do this? I suggest a process with three parts: (1) each person letting the other know clearly what they are sensitive to, so each can stop poking at the other's wounds; (2) all parties recognizing that these sensitive wounds are old stuff, and that they are less about the other(s) and more about themselves; (3) each person responding differently, generally the opposite of the usual or established reflexive response—be assertive instead of withdrawing, stop accommodating but instead be clear about needs, controlling anger but using the anger as information about unmet needs or boundary violations. This is about moving toward; the partners saying to one another what they couldn't say to their parents when they were children. By stopping the rewounding process and responding differently in the present, each person, over time, begins to heal the wounds of the past.

What to Do

Look for and ask what each person is most sensitive to—micromanaging, dismissal, lack of appreciation, criticism, or neglect. Educate the couple or family about these negative loops and the ways of breaking them. And when the loops are recreated in the session, stop the process and help them be aware of what is unfolding.

3. Vision

Sometimes a conflict has to do with the future—I want to live in New York City; I want to get a small farm out in the country and grow our food; I want to have three kids; I want to have none and live in South America. Sometimes it is about the everyday life in the relationship—I need time by myself on weekends to work on my projects; I want to see my parents on the weekends; I want to have dinner parties on Friday nights; I want to stay home on Fridays and get pizza and watch a movie.

Attending to clients' "visions" is about determining priorities and what it means to be a couple or family. While poor communication and emotional wounds make working together all the more challenging, often this obstacle stands on its own. It is about compatibility and both partners adjusting to the typical personal changes that arise with aging and life experiences. For example, those entering their midlife crisis or retirement often are acutely aware that time is running out, and so they push for significant change—starting a new career, moving closer to their family, wanting more intimacy, having more common interests. The hard questions are often: Do we share enough things in common to make this work? What is the one thing I can only get from you that is enough to override everything else? The couple or family members talk about being at opposite poles or resenting the change the other wants or is unwilling to make. These are the difficult conversations that need to happen.

What to Do

Frame the problem as one of differing visions. Help them define their individual visions, be assertive in stating them, see if they can reach win–win compromises, and ask hard questions about bottom lines and what-ifs. Help them move through the decision process.

What these obstacles have in common is that each, in its own way, keeps couples and families from successfully solving their problems or moving forward in their lives together. By looking for these obstacles at the start and helping them see what you, as the outsider, see that they often cannot, you reframe their concerns—not about whose reality is right, who has a problem, who is being unreasonable or insensitive—but about the stuckness itself. You step out of playing judge and sorting facts and instead help them focus on learning skills and changing the process.

Finally, because we are talking about relationships, all these obstacles can characterize breakdowns in the therapeutic relationship. Communication can go awry; emotional wounds translate into transference and countertransference reactions, and differing visions easily apply to differing expectations about the therapy process or the treatment plan. Look for these obstacles here as well.

Finally, what obstacles do you most struggle with when you look back over your personal relationships? What are your emotional wounds? Where does communication break down? Is your vision compatible with your partner's? What do you need to focus on and change most?

CHAPTER 25

Children, Families, and Therapy

Children are frequently part of the therapy mix in some form—as the presenting problem as individuals or as part of a family in play or talking therapy, or in some combination. Likely your skills with children will depend on whether you took courses in child therapy or did child work as part of your internships and fieldwork, as well as your personal experience with children as a parent, coach, or teacher. Regardless of your starting point, integrating children into therapy, treating them at different ages with different needs, is a subset of clinical treatment that can be intimidating even for more experienced clinicians.

To help you navigate these waters, here's an overview of the different roles, challenges, and options you might have when working with children.

Tagalong Kids

The parents arrive at their first session with their three-month-old baby, who is in a car seat and is, fortunately, sleeping. Or they come with a preschooler or a gaggle of school-age kids—the babysitter canceled at the last minute, and there wasn't time to take them home before coming in. The kids are not there as clients but tagalongs. Your challenge is accommodation and logistics. The baby may be a problem—ideally, you want and ask the parents ahead of time to find a way to come in together as a couple sans baby—and now, if you're lucky, the parents are working around the baby's usual nap time. But it's a baby, and you never know what may erupt. A crying baby can keep you from gaining any forward momentum, dilute those emotional, critical moments, or provide the parent, who really didn't want to come, with a good excuse to avoid talking to you. This happens; you need to think on your feet and adjust. If the baby takes over the session, ask if one of the parents can take charge, take the baby to the waiting room, and then switch midpoint in the session.

Although less eruptive and unpredictable perhaps, the preschooler too can be a distraction. Proactive parents will bring toys or, better yet, games on their phones that the child can play with. Or, if the child is old enough, you can give him or her some paper and crayons to draw with. (If you are seeing a lot of children, it helps to have a child-size table in your office for them.) Although it's easy to talk over the child's head, parents will often worry, as they should, that the emotional tone in the room will affect the child and inhibit not only what they say but how they say it. You need to monitor and be sensitive to the emotional climate in the room and even have the parents take turns or check in with the child periodically: "How are you doing on the game, Sara? Are you okay?"

Finally, if the clients show up with the kid gaggle, the gaggle can usually be left in the waiting room with their computers or phones and art supplies. If you or the parents sense it's getting too quiet or too loud, that's usually a sign that someone needs to check on the kids. Often one of the children will bang on the office door, and the parent needs to guide the child back to the waiting room, reboot the computer, ask an older sibling to be in charge until the session is over, and if they're good, they'll all get ice cream after.

Children in Couple Therapy

By definition, children are not physically part of couple therapy, but that doesn't mean that children are not mentally in the room as the couple's initial concern. Many couple therapists have had the experience of couples presenting with child issues, only to shift focus in the third session and talk about the real concern, namely issues in their intimate relationship. The child's problems were a comfortable way station that bought the couple time to check you out and feel settled and safe before marching into the more contentious territory and their real agenda.

When children are the couple's primary focus, the parents' concerns can take several forms. Parents of fourteen-year-olds, for example, may seek therapy because they fear their teen may have a budding eating disorder. The teen refuses to come in or even respond to the parents' concerns, and so the parents are seeking information about the disorder—ideas about when to seek medical consultation and tips about ways to initiate this conversation with their daughter at home. In addition to struggling with their own lack of sleep and irritability, parents of newborns may be unsure how to help their three-year-old who suddenly feels dethroned and is throwing tantrums.

Other parents struggle to adapt their parenting styles to their growing children. The five-year-old who could be picked up and placed in time-out when cranky is now a teen taller than his mother; when he quickly becomes defiant when asked to take out the garbage, his mother is at a loss for what to do. Often your role in such cases is education and skill training, helping the parents understand their child's changing needs and how to best communicate and behaviorally respond.

But for many parents who come as a couple, the presenting issue is their differences in parenting styles and differing visions of the role of children in the family and how these differences should be treated. Usually, the source of their differences lies in their reactions to the parenting they received as children: The parent who was neglected as a child is now forever attentive; the child of abusive parents fears turning into his father and is overly accommodating. But differences can reflect different values—one parent believes that children and family time should be the primary everyday focus, while the other feels that the couple needs to have more time for themselves. The clash in values can often reflect conflicting cultural and ethnic foundations.

At the most extreme form, these parents are polarized: One parent is easy because the other is too strict; one is too strict because the other is too easy. When seeing such parents together, there is a feeling in the room of an ongoing power struggle, that the couple is playing courtroom and trying to have you play judge to decide who is right and who is not.

This polarization can be harmful to children in several ways. One is that some children learn how to split the parents, play one against the other, and make requests of the easy parent when the other is not around. Not only does this behavior fuel the parents' conflict, but the child learns to be manipulative and entitled and will likely become a hellion when he becomes a teen. Another by-product is that the children get a distorted, one-dimensional view of each parent—my dad is accommodating, my mom strict—shaping their expectations about adult relationships and providing poor role modeling for their own parenting. Perhaps the biggest concern is that such children are living at home in a constant state of tension, spawning individual anxiety or acting out through sibling rivalry.

The parents' differences become the starting point for treatment: bypass playing courtroom and move them toward developing a unified plan. How to do this will depend on your clinical models. For example, if your model is psychodynamic or Bowenian, you may explore the couple's upbringing and relationship with their parents. If it is structural, you may emphasize the need to have a clear hierarchy; if it is cognitive-behavioral, ask about their thoughts about parenting and about ways they respond when problems arise and provide behavioral homework assignments that help the couple support rather than undermine each other.

Children in Family Therapy

Sometimes one or both parents are requesting family therapy. The couple is getting divorced, the children are suffering in their own ways, and the parents want a safe forum to explain to the children what will unfold. Or Grandpa passed away, the children are struggling, and the parents don't know how to talk with them about his death. Or there's a new boyfriend in the home, and although the younger daughter loves all the attention she receives, the older son feels dethroned and competitive and battles with him daily.

With other clients, it's you, the clinician, who asks that the entire family come in, perhaps even including important extended-family members, such as grandparents. Such total family sessions allow you to observe all the interactional processes as they unfold in the room; you can quickly gather important assessment information and connect with each family member, minimizing the danger of those left out undermining the treatment process.

And yes, such total family sessions can understandably seem overwhelming, especially if you're new at doing them. If you decide to see the entire family, you may want to have the support of a cotherapist. But because family therapy is less about everyone in the room and more about thinking in terms of family dynamics—patterns and history, projections, and communication—you have options; you can decide what you need to be comfortable. Instead of seeing the entire family at the start, see the parents alone first to assess their relationship and define goals. Or see the entire family, but do breakouts: a third of the session with the parents, a third with the child or sibs, a third together. Decide at the front end what works best for you.

Whatever mix and number of family members you eventually settle on, take the time to establish rapport with each child. Ask about their world—their hobbies, interests, friends. Match their voice tone and vocabulary level. School-age children, and certainly teens, are verbal enough to describe their emotions and problems—ask what they would like to see changed the most. And then do what you would do with couples—stop them from arguing about whose reality is right, change the language of anger to one of worry, help them negotiate possible solutions that they can agree on and try out at home, ask the hard questions to discover where the family gets stuck solving their own problems so it can move forward.

Sibling Groups

Sometimes it is helpful to see siblings together without the parents, especially when a younger family member feels intimidated by the process. I remember a case where the three children—five, seven, and nine—witnessed their mother being shot by her boyfriend. The mother was in rehab, the children stayed with the grandparents, and all were traumatized. Although the seven- and nine-year-olds could talk about their feelings—guilt, fear, confusion—the little five-year-old sister was shut down. But in her brothers' presence, she could hear, and they could verbalize what she could not say. She would nod her head and, with their comforting presence and modeling, she was able over time to begin to speak for herself.

Individual Children and Parents

Tom has been getting into fights at school; Denice isn't sleeping and always complains of stomachaches. The parents request that you see the child for treatment; again there are options.

One is to start by seeing the parents and child together for the initial session. (I once had a family in which the parents literally dropped their eight-year-old off at the front of the building while they waited in the car; talk about "fix-my-kid" expectations.) Take a few minutes to connect with the parents and the child. Explain your role to the child—that you are a "worry doctor" or that you are like the guidance counselor at school and that you help children and parents with their feelings and problems. Ask the parents to describe their concerns to the child so he knows why he is there. Seeing that the parents are comfortable with you will help the child feel the same. Once you sense that the child has settled, you can then ask him if he is willing to play or talk with you for a few minutes while his parents wait close by in the waiting room.

But my first-session preference is to see the parents together without the child. Why? Because it allows you to get a more detailed history—the scope of their concerns, what they've tried, what's worked, what hasn't—that the parents might not feel comfortable openly sharing with the child present or that doing so would eat up too much time. But more important, you can drill down and make sure they are on the same page. If not, if they disagree about the problem, are polarized, or can't work together as a team, we need to hold off on seeing the child until they can reach some consensus.

Finally, you can often bypass seeing the child at all by seeing the parents alone. It is time-efficient; you potentially sidestep any need to build the relationship so the child feels comfortable with a stranger in a strange environment doing strange things. Once you can visualize the behavioral patterns in the home—you say *x*, she says *y*; you do *x*, she does *y*—you can empower the parents to essentially become the child's therapists. Just as the air traffic controller explains to the unskilled emergency pilot how to land the plane, by giving the parents specific, clear directions about what to say and how to respond, you can help them change the dysfunctional patterns within the family. Have the parents try the approach for a couple of weeks, fine-tune it, and see if it makes a difference. If the child's behavior is still not better, it's time to bring the child in to separate the family dynamics from the child's possible inner struggles.

Individual Children

Just as you can decide how to use family therapy, you can also choose how to use your work with the individual child. As we just discussed, you may primarily work through the parents—provide suggestions at the start, help them make behavioral changes in the home, and then reevaluate. Or you reverse the order—focus on the child for a few sessions to assess and then provide the parents feedback about what changes to make in the home. Or you may decide to see an individual for treatment—working, for example, with a child who has been traumatized by abuse.

Here, as you are potentially doing in all therapy, you are taking on the role of the ideal parent to protect against triggering old wounds and hopefully to heal them. What is different about play therapy is that you are using play as a medium to help the child express her emotions and, with your guidance, see them in a new light. You will undoubtedly use play as your primary medium if the child is young. With a child who is ten or eleven, you are in a transitional zone: Some ten- or eleven-year-olds will still respond best to straight play therapy, while for others play is the background for conversations (playing checkers or card games, for example, as you talk), or you may move directly to conversations.

You'll need to explore and experiment, but again keep your options in mind from the start.

Adolescents in Therapy

Some teens come to therapy because they want therapy. They tell their parents that they are unhappy or anxious, have broken up with a boyfriend and are grieving, or struggle with their sexual identity. They probably have a preference for a male or a female therapist. Still, they are motivated, and if you are a good listener, can be the unparent, and can avoid overreacting or loading them down with lectures and advice, they will open up. Adolescents, after all, still need adult guidance; they just don't often want it from their parents because they're individuating, and privacy is important.

But many other teens are dragged into treatment by their frustrated or worried parents. Sixteen-year-old Teresa, for example, accompanies her parents to an initial family session. The parents start by railing about her boyfriend; her grades are dropping, and she's got an "attitude." Watch what happens. If Teresa can push back despite being overrun, she's got some grit—good to go. Step up to shape the process—keep it from getting too emotional, press the family to be clear, ask the hard questions, and help them advance toward win–win compromises.

If Teresa says nothing and stares off into space, you need to stop the process. She is getting emotionally beaten up, and you condone it with your silence. Rather than creating the safety she needs, she sees you as just another adult giving her a hard time. Time to show leadership. Ask Teresa if she would mind your talking with her alone. She will usually nod in agreement; you send the parents to the waiting room. Once they leave, you turn to Teresa and say in a gentle voice, "Wow, is this what they always do?" Teresa will now roll her eyes and nod her head.

Your goal for the rest of the session is to draw Teresa out and create rapport, helping her see that you are not just another adult who rants at her about her life. Help her define what she would like to change at home in her family—that she wants her parents to get off her back, to stop them from treating her like a child, to realize that she can make good decisions and is not as oblivious or incompetent as they think she is. This is great; you now have a therapeutic contract with her. Your challenge now is to bring together the warring factions: connect the parents' concerns—her grades and attitude—with what Teresa wants—her parents to be less micromanaging. Developing a plan that addresses the parents' concerns and those of Teresa becomes the focus of therapy.

The theme here is that, like other areas of therapy, your role in working with children of all ages comes with challenges; the key is getting the training and support you need to be proactive, planful, and confident. But, like those other areas, you always have options. Therapy is not like repairing a computer or a broken pipe. It is flexible; you are free to build around your comfort zones and strengths.

And if you do, you will become the best therapist you can be.

CHAPTER 26

Working with Play

If navigating how to fit children into the therapy process can seem challenging, the mega-notion of doing play therapy can seem even harder. Maybe it's because you simply don't know what you're doing and lack the skills; or no, to be honest, you really don't enjoy children and prefer the world of adults and talking. Or it's not about kids—you love them, especially your own—but seeing kids at work and at home is just . . . too many kids; you need a break and a job where you can talk with adults.

If it's about skills, it's time to get some training. There are plenty of options out there. You may be able to connect with Allie, your work colleague who has been doing play therapy for a thousand years, and ask if you can sit in on a few sessions or have her coach you through a few cases. But if there is no Allie, you can sign up for workshops, look at videos, and seek out conferences. Be proactive; tell your supervisor what you need to do the good job you were hired for. Through this training exploration, you can decide how much of this type of work you want to do.

And if you decide that you enjoy working with children (or if you really don't have much choice), you can determine how you want to use play in your work. If, for example, you are seeing a five-year-old who is clearly anxious—chewing on her clothes or has separation anxiety each morning when her father tries to drop her off at school—you may first try working through the parents, coaching them on ways to help her with her anxiety. If that isn't working, switch to play therapy as the form of treatment.

What do you need to do play therapy? Most often, not much. Crayons, paints, drawing paper, clay. Some blocks, a playhouse, people figures to live in the house, some cars, trucks, an ambulance perhaps. Puppets, animal figures, toy soldiers, some Legos: toys that stimulate imaginative play. For younger children, board games like Uno, Candy Land, and Chutes and Ladders; board games can provide more grounding in the present than video games, which can too quickly mentally sweep them up. For older ones, checkers, Battleship, Risk, and Sorry can be used to build rapport and as background for talking. Get a deck of cards, hook up a mini basketball net over your office door, and use a Nerf ball for the basketball. Most of what you need to get started can be found at a big-box store or at garage sales, or borrowed from friends whose kids have outgrown their toys. Set out the art supplies and games in your office where the children can see and choose from them.

But once children reach the age of ten to twelve, they often enter a transition zone. A few may still engage in imaginative play, but others will see it as babyish. Here drawing or playing Uno while talking about their parents' divorce provides just enough distraction to keep them from feeling overwhelmed. Yet other children in this age range—those who are more comfortable and verbal around adults—need no props; they are happy to sit in on family sessions to express their worries.

If you don't want to use play as a treatment method, you can use it as an assessment tool. You ask eight-year-old Matt to draw a picture of his family. Dad is twice as tall as everyone else, and off in the corner of the page the rest of the family is huddled together—maybe a good time to talk with the parents and especially the dad about ways to improve his standing in the family. Or the five-year-old who chews on her clothes doesn't play out a scene from her home life, as you thought she would, but instead creates a scene with dolls where she is at school and her "mean" teacher is yelling at her to stop fidgeting in her seat. You may decide to continue with play therapy to help her manage her anxiety, or you may reach out to the parents about talking with the teacher, or both.

But while you're working through these larger issues of play therapy theory and techniques and the role of play therapy in your treatment plan, don't forget to consider the family context. Here you need to make sure the parents are on board. This is about mapping out expectations. Are they able to see it as a form of treatment rather than just play ("All my son said you did last week was play Candy Land with him for an hour"), or would it be better to focus on their parental skills? Are they and you willing to take the time needed to engage in what may be a slower process? Is there any danger of the child's status as the family problem being reinforced through this individual focus? Just as some adults use one form of therapy more effectively than another, so do children and families.

The bottom line is that play therapy with children is another approach, modality, and clinical choice. Again it is flexible enough as a medium that you and the family have options, that you can adapt it not only to the particular needs of a child and the family, but also to your own style and strengths.

CHAPTER 27

Time to Check In

The practice of checking in is about pausing, stepping back, taking the pulse, and surveying the landscape. It keeps you, the client, and the process from running on autopilot, driven by routine and comfort. It's also preventative, allowing you to catch potential problems before they erupt into big ones that can cause the treatment to stall or the client to disappear. There are several ways to use check-ins. Here's a good sampler.

Check-Ins during the Session

We previously discussed the importance of you and the client staying in lockstep as you move through the session, shifting your focus and periodically stepping back to take the emotional temperature in the room—both forms of checking in throughout the session. When you explain your overall clinical approach, make an interpretation, frame the client's problem in a new way, you want to get a solid yes, either by a nodding of the head or a verbal agreement. When providing information, you want to make sure the client is attentive. If you get solid yeses all the way down the line, if the client remains engaged, you don't have to worry about objections when it's time to propose your preliminary treatment plan or set the next appointment.

But if you don't—your interpretation is countered by a confused look, your reframe is met with a weak "I guess," or you realize that your "lecturette" has gone on too long and you're losing your audience—you want to stop. You've fallen out of step; the emotional climate has changed; there's a problem in the room. If you don't address it, you'll be dealing with yes, buts or "I need to check my calendar and get back to you later" at the end of the session. Throughout your sessions, this checking for agreement and engagement is what you want to do to prevent any accumulating resistance.

Check-Ins for Accountability

Dan agreed to talk with his mom about her rule about gaming during the school week; Eleanor said that she would set an appointment with her psychiatrist to double-check her meds; to stop the snipping and snapping at each other about money, Jamal and Terese planned to have a meeting to create a budget that worked for both of them; Ray, a writer, said he would leave you a voice mail message telling you how many words he had written that day. You check in with Dan, Eleanor, Jamal, and Terese at the top of the next session: Did you do ____________? How'd it go? If Ray fails to leave a message, you send him one.

Certainly, following up with clients about homework is essential to find out if what you suggested and what they agreed to do worked. Like staying in lockstep, follow-up prevents problems from going undetected and accumulating. But it is also about accountability—making sure they did or are doing what they said they would do. There's a reason AA or NA members check in with their sponsors during the week—it's challenging to change well-ingrained patterns and habits; there's a natural internal resistance. Knowing you'll report to someone and having someone look over your shoulder pushes you forward. It's why Pinocchio had Jiminy Cricket sitting on his.

Check-Ins Every Few Sessions

Five or six sessions are a good number. This check-in can be a two-liner said near the end of a session: "So I'm just checking in. I just want to make sure that you feel that what we've been doing so far has been helpful; whether there's anything we have not yet talked about that you want to talk about or whether there is anything we need to do differently?"

You are again checking for lockstep, the relationship's emotional climate, and the process from a few steps further back. By checking in, you're essentially conveying several messages at the same time: that this is your therapy, you're the consumer, and I want to make sure you are getting what you need; that you have a voice; this is a collaborative process, feel free to speak up; finally, you're saying, "Let's avoid going on autopilot, falling into a routine, doing what we do because we do it."

Client Check-Ins

Tara wants to work on her zero-to-60 anger. Carl's panic attacks seem to arise out of nowhere. You say to each of them: "I'd like you to check in with yourself every hour or two. On a scale of one to ten, one being that you're flatlined and emotionally okay and ten that you're becoming psychotic, see how you are doing. When you get to a three or four, are feeling irritable, worried, or out of sorts, ask yourself, 'What's going on? Is there a problem I need to fix? Is there something I need to do to change my mood?' "

This is about clients checking in with themselves and assessing their own emotional state. It's a powerful therapeutic tool. Folks who quickly escalate usually have a hard time catching the subtle buildup of anger or anxiety and, once it gets to a six or more, it's difficult for them to rein these emotions in. By asking them to do check-ins regularly, they, over time, become more attuned to what is happening. By catching this buildup of emotion, they have the space to proactively reduce it and begin to rewire their brains.

Check In with Yourself

This may be the most important check-in of all: Checking in with yourself, stepping back from the grind or monotony of your work or your life and taking your own pulse. Are you and your life in lockstep? Is there anything you need to change in your professional or personal life? Are your goals the same ones you had six months ago, a year ago? Are you feeling bored, is your life too routinized, do you need to run your life differently? Is too much of you getting left out of you?

How are you doing?

CHAPTER 28

First Aid for Those Awful Sessions

The session with Bill is rocking along—you're sipping your coffee, nodding your head—and then you comment that what he said to his partner sounds similar to what he had described his father often saying to his mother. But then—bam! The therapeutic train suddenly derails. Bill stomps out of the room. Shell-shocked, you can't decide whether to let him go or chase him down the hall.

Or suddenly six-year-old Eric collapses into a full-blown tantrum while his father, hands on hips, stands over him yelling, "Stop! Just stop this minute!" By the time the smoke clears and Eric exhausts himself, you're ten minutes late for your next client.

Or maybe there isn't any drama—no one stomps out or collapses—but instead, you're left at the end of the session wondering if anyone is coming back. Marie left seeming annoyed, maybe, you think, because you didn't come down harder on her partner about her drinking. Or you took the bold step of confronting ever-reliable weekly-session Ann about her pattern of making excuses for her mother's emotionally abusive behavior. Now, for no apparent reason, she's unsure what her work schedule looks like and will have to circle back about setting another appointment. Hmmm . . .

This happens to us all—those explosive sessions or awful sessions where things erupt or turn out at the end way different from what you had planned. And yes, it can rattle your self-confidence or cause you to stare at your bedroom ceiling at 3:00 A.M. This is the downside of working with people instead of with computers—their unpredictability, all those emotions. But there are first-aid steps you can take; think of them as Step 1 and Step 2.

Step 1

Step 1 is first aid—what to do in the session when things go out of control. It is more about not feeding the emotional fire than trying to put it out. If a client is going into a rage, remain calm, listen, talk in a soft voice: Anything you say at this point can quickly add fuel to the fire. Skip the mini-lecture about anger or trying to explain to Bill why you mentioned his father. Bill's rational brain is off-line and can't process information. Save your information or your explanation for later.

And if Bill stomps out, do you chase him down? In my early days, I did, probably because I was flustered and didn't know what else to do. I stopped doing that a long time ago. Most clients, I realized, stomp off because they are emotionally flooded, can't handle any more input, and need the time and space to cool off. Once they did, they would usually circle back on their own. But if you are seriously worried about your clients' state after leaving, or if they have not circled back, call or text them to check in so they don't feel abandoned and so you don't remain anxious. And obviously, if you believe they could harm themselves or someone else, take immediate action—talk to your supervisor, call the police.

And what about melting-down Eric? See what unfolds and what the dad can do. Is Eric settling down; is dad? Or is dad ramping up and yelling at Eric more? Likely they are replicating a well-established problem and pattern, which is a good opportunity to teach skills in vitro. There is no need to take over, but instead, lower the temperature by coaching the dad on how to help his child.

Of course, let's not forget those poor clients twiddling their thumbs when you're running over. If possible, give your next client a heads-up via the front desk person or a text or step out of the room for a moment; this is about courtesy. If you can't, many apologies are needed at the start of their session.

A Larger Pattern?

But if melting-down clients and running late are more than occasional events, you need to wonder why. Sure, it may be the profile of your client population, but more likely, part of the problem lies with you. Maybe you're not tracking the process close enough—noticing how Bill always becomes anxious whenever you ask about his father or not catching the early signs that Eric is getting agitated. If so, you want to practice paying attention to any emotional shifts and address them then and there—asking your Bills or Erics about how they were feeling or why they seemed upset. Similarly, you may need to work on pacing and watching the clock: not raising strong emotions too near the end of the session but instead waiting to the next one; not overwhelming clients by giving them too much information too quickly at the close of the session, leaving little time to explain or process. Step back and see if you can uncover the underlying problems.

Step 2

Step 2 is about mopping up. So, you don't chase Bill down the hall, but you follow up with a text or call an hour or two later. And you certainly want to do the same for Marie and Ann. If you are worried about their parting reactions, don't just fret; act. Call, text, or email Marie and Ann and voice your concerns: "I know our session yesterday was emotionally difficult. I'm wondering if you felt upset because ____________ [I wasn't more confrontational with your partner, that you felt I was being critical . . .]." Say what you think the client may be thinking. Offer to talk about it more via a phone conversation or at the next session. On the other hand, if you are less concerned and feel comfortable that they will circle back on their own, wait until the next session to follow up. But follow up with them early in the next session to underscore your concern and have enough time to process: "I've been concerned about how you felt at the end of our last session. Did you feel ____________?"

Reaching out in this way is often healing; you are likely doing what other important people in their lives never do—showing concern about tears in the relationship by openly talking about them and trying to repair them. Likely Marie or Ann will appreciate your comments and efforts and respond accordingly. Or they may not, but you've done your best.

And again, if clients who leave sessions disappointed or upset is part of a larger pattern for you, the question to yourself is why. It may be about not staying in lockstep and noticing when you and the client are out of sync, about time management and leaving enough time in sessions to mop up around objections and concerns, or about missing transference cues and triggering emotional wounds. Talk to your supervisor and, if possible, tape sessions to better track the unfolding microprocess.

These awful sessions are painful but are also opportunities to learn. Treat yourself kindly; figure out the moral of the story.

CHAPTER 29

When a Client Is in Crisis

In the last chapter, we discussed those awful, unexpected crisis sessions that can be difficult to navigate. Here we're talking about crises outside the session, those in clients' everyday lives that spark their reaching out to you. Crises can erupt for a variety of reasons, but not all crises are created equally—different reasons mean different drivers, which in turn means a different response from you. To help you map out what you might encounter, here is a quick survey of the most common types and guidelines on how to respond.

The Crisis Event

Shanelle, a long-term client, has used therapy as a monthly way of checking in, bouncing off ideas about handling a problem. You have always seen her as having a great base of coping skills. But midmonth, she unexpectedly contacts you: her daughter had been raped, and she feels like she is falling apart. For other clients, it may be getting the news that they have Stage IV cancer, that a parent has suddenly died after what seemed like a case of the flu, or that their house was blown away by a tornado.

Regardless of the circumstances, these folks are dealing with actual life events that automatically spin them into shock, grief, and uncertainty about what to do. They are looking to you for support and guidance. You're doing trauma intervention—being the person they can vent to and help them figure out the next steps or put things into a larger perspective. They reach out because of their connection to you, that safe person to turn to who is outside their family and free of those emotional entanglements. Your goal is to guide them through this period of pain, confusion, and loss.

And so, you do; you become their crisis center—empathize with and support them, help them think through ways to talk with others close to them who are dealing with the same crisis, provide resources, check in and make sure they are okay. This is about human-to-human contact, a verbal and emotional therapeutic hug, a pat on the back. Your message is that this is awful, but you can get through this, and I'm here to help you.

The Overwhelmed Client

Your client Stephen is texting you five times an hour. He just heard that there are cutbacks on his job and feels overwhelmed and panicky; he needs to talk. You're not sure what he's looking for, but you know that this is not the first time he's fallen into this state.

As discussed in the last chapter, your response to Stephen is in two steps. Step 1: Lower the emotional temperature and help him calm down. You let him vent; you show empathy and bring perspective; you help him get his rational brain back online.

Step 2: Mop up, and learn the moral of the story. Once Stephen settles, because you've helped him gain perspective or because he finds out he isn't going to get fired, it is time to circle back. Time to deconstruct; move out of the content of the job and to his coping process and panicky reaction: What triggered his feeling so overwhelmed? Could he tell that his anxiety was building and running through his brain? Is there something else he could have done if he couldn't reach you?

The danger here is that if you only do Step 1 and help Stephen calm down but skip Step 2, he will grow more and more dependent on you to help him cope, and his ability to manage his anxiety will go down, not up. While he is ready to put this crisis behind him once he has settled, your goal is to wean him off you and help him develop the emotional-regulation skills he needs to lean on himself; they are the skills that Shanelle has but Stephen, for whatever reason, lacks. You clearly talk about his need to develop these skills; you look for and address any resistance. To break his crisis pattern, you want to get him on board.

Seeking Therapy to Put Out Fires

Yuan has left you a half dozen phone messages. He found you online, said that he and his partner had a big fight; she left, and he needs to talk to someone now! He will try to convince his partner to come in with him to see you, hoping you can help persuade her not to leave. But if she refuses, maybe he could give you her phone number: Could you call and talk to her, let her know he called you, and maybe change her mind?

It's Friday afternoon; you get a call from Alex. "Hi," he says. "I got your name from my attorney. I'm calling because I'm scheduled to go to court next week about some misunderstanding. My attorney suggested that it would be helpful if I could get a psychological evaluation to help bolster my case. I realize it's Friday afternoon, but I'm free anytime on Monday. Wondering if I could come in and we could chat and, if you could write up something to give to my attorney by Tuesday, that would be great."

Yes, Yuan and Alex are in crisis, but their crises differ from Stephen's panicky texts. Yuan and Alex are looking for a firefighter—someone to put out the current crisis that is overwhelming them. You may explain to Yuan that your job is not to take sides in couple therapy, nor are you comfortable calling his partner, but you would be happy to see them together if they want a safe place to discuss and work through their issues. You may explain to Alex that you need to understand what he and his attorney are actually looking for and that because a proper assessment is more than a one-session "chat," you wouldn't be able to meet his deadline. If this assessment is something he might need after the court date, he's welcome to circle back, and you could discuss it further. You're resetting their expectations.

While Yuan and Alex's emotions and needs are understandable, it's hard not to feel like they are trying to manipulate you for their own ends. Fortunately, these situations don't happen that often, but you can feel rattled and unsure about how to respond when they do. Talk to your supervisor or colleagues in advance to avoid responding on the fly and to lower your anxiety. Get their input so you can develop your own policy and response.

Crisis Families

If you work in community mental health or are allied to your local social service system, you will probably become familiar with those families who seem to always go in and out of crises. The triggers will likely vary—the electricity has been cut off, a letter from the landlord about overdue rent payments arrives, a child is getting in trouble at school, or there is some health emergency. Life is good when everything is going well, but when bad stuff happens, the family is overwhelmed. They reach out to you or your agency to bail them out—asking for money to pay the electric bill or rent, someone to talk to the principal about the child and provide support around the health crisis. Unlike Shanelle's crisis, these crises are not one-time events but a seemingly endless series of problems with breaks in between.

Like the others, they feel overwhelmed for good reasons and are doing the best they can. They also likely have additional long-standing stressors, such as poverty, poor coping skills, or mental illness. But if this pattern of falling into crisis is, in fact, a pattern, the clinical question is: What do they need to manage their lives better?

Often the parents grew up in similar crisis-driven environments where they learned to see life as one darn thing after another and to look to others to help put out fires. Unfortunately, they didn't know how to be proactive rather than reactive, address problems before they reach the crisis state, and develop those good habits that prevent problems from arising in the first place. Instead, they've fallen into a pattern where they weather the crisis, feel exhausted but relieved, but never learn the lessons that the situation can teach.

Your challenge is selling them on the idea that crises are not inevitable if they can be more proactive. Here you or a case manager may check in with the family twice a week to track signs of any impending problems and encourage them to take action—contact the school when they receive the first note from the teacher or the rental office about overdue rent; bring Grandma to the doctor when she first complains about pain. They will need your support and encouragement to break out of their all-or-nothing thinking.

Too Many Crisis Clients in Your Caseload?

If you're not working in a crisis-oriented setting such as emergency services but find that many of your clients seem to be in crisis, you may want to step back and ask yourself why. It may simply reflect the population that your agency serves. But if that's not the case, the culprit is likely to be a lack of skills. Perhaps you viewed Stephen's bursts of anxiety as situational rather than as something more pervasive. Or when your client Roger made offhand references to suicide, you tried to smooth over his comments with suggestions about doing some couple therapy with his wife or about increasing his medications.

This is about missing cues because you don't have good treatment maps or about mentally sweeping anxiety-provoking situations under the rug. If you have either of these shortcomings, it's time to get some training to build up your skills so you don't feel overwhelmed. This is, of course, not only about helping your clients, but ultimately about helping yourself.

CHAPTER 30

Working with Clients Who Are Different from You

I remember reading Monica McGoldrick's *Ethnicity and Family Therapy* when it came out over 40 years ago. With its chapters on Italian, Jewish, and Irish families and their unique cultures, it seemed to open the door to the notion that clients may actually be different from us, and we, as therapists, need to consider these differences in our work. Of course, since then, our awareness and sensitivity have exponentially grown. We (and she) have moved beyond those predominantly white families and clients to try improving our models and our work with the full array of people who come to our clinics and with clients facing unique stressors and challenges—immigrants, for example, from wartorn countries carrying within them not only their culture but their trauma.

And we've expanded our perspective as well, looking beyond family life to question and grapple with the subtle but devastating ways our societal culture has impacted the psyche and everyday lives of, say, African Americans in this country, or with our understanding of how someone living with a physical disability is faced with coping in a society that is often uncaring, unnoticing, even at times hostile. And in recent years, we've learned to stop thinking about gender and sexuality as belonging to X or Y camps but to think in terms of a broader spectrum.

While we've come a long way in our sensitivity and should be proud of how far we've come as a society and a profession, our awareness has made what we do seem more complex. A number of things I have learned occur to me when I think about the way these differences impact the therapy process.

They're Uncomfortable

I recently met with a student from India, and his opening question in our first session was, "Have you worked with a lot of Indian students?" I answered his question honestly: "Yes, I have worked with several Indian students in the past few years." But the question that immediately popped into my head was: Why is he asking that question? And I immediately knew the answer: He was asking, "Are you able to understand me even though I am different from you?" This initial dialogue was about what we would call rapport, but what he might call feeling safe.

While he was forthright about his concerns, I can easily imagine that many clients are not as brave. They may be intimidated by the unfamiliar process, or their culture makes them shy with professionals, or they have a long history of dealing with public agencies and have learned that they have little say over who they may be assigned and need to accept who they get.

But if they don't speak up because they feel they can't, I believe we need to. You create safety not by ignoring the elephant in the room but by pointing to it, by getting differences on the table, by giving clients the space to define themselves: "Because I'm not Muslim," you say. "Help me understand how your religion [or your culture, your disability, your gender] factors into your life, so I better understand how it may impact our work. What is it that you feel is important for me to understand about you and your culture, condition, or identification?" And then you listen deeply to what they say next.

By asking such questions, you are letting clients know that the differences between us are not just okay to talk about but necessary to talk about. By listening to their answers, you're conveying that this is an important concern not only to them but also to you.

You're Uncomfortable

Of course, the other side of this relationship equation is you—your own reactions and anxiety. If you are just starting out, the differences between you and your clients may add to the performance pressures you already feel. You want to be sensitive and do it right, but the danger is that you walk on eggshells, give up your leadership, and become too passive.

Such reactions are understandable, but resist the pressure and urge. Yes, you want to be sensitive—for example, be careful with your use of language when talking with someone who is highly religious—but you don't want to overaccommodate either, for example, having bible verses to quote at the ready to build a connection. Such watering down of your clinical style not only makes you less effective, but also prevents clients from being able to honestly decide whether the relationship is a good fit.

Differences Are Part of the Problem

But sometimes the differences are not between you and the client but between them and partners or family members, and these differences bring them into therapy. Here we can think of situations where one partner has made a recent religious conversion, and the other is reeling from the sudden change in climate, values, and priorities. Or it's about political differences—the liberal couple who united around climate change or tax relief for the poor are now battling over whether to install a heat pump and insulation or whether the poor need to start taking more responsibility for improving themselves. Or teens who announce that they want to change their gender and the parents who are trying to be supportive, while at the same time struggling to wrap their heads around the disclosure and manage their anxiety.

Often in these situations, the clients are hoping you'll play judge—clearly say who's right or wrong or at least lean to their side and be the voice of reason that will finally convince the other person that she's crazy or to get her to leave them alone. You obviously don't want to take on this role or get into the weeds about God's word, climate change, or the effects of hormone injections. Instead, you want to shape the process so that each person is heard. You want to deepen the conversation by asking how their changed thinking came about. Most of all, you want to draw out and acknowledge the underlying problem they likely have in common: a sense of loss, the worry that the differences will become a divide and that their mutual futures are forever altered. Only by doing this can they get beyond the facts and figures of the issues and move together toward a satisfying resolution.

Differences are yet another potential pothole on the therapeutic path. You can work with clients to fill them in or at least agree to walk around them so you can continue walking together. But sometimes what you do won't be enough. Despite your best efforts, the Indian student doesn't feel safe and so doesn't continue; the couple expected you to decide who was right and who was wrong and when you don't, they think therapy is a waste of time; the parents or teen hear what you say about the underlying problem, but they dismiss the idea as soon as they leave your office.

It's okay; you've done your job, been sensitive, and addressed their differences. Once again, you've done the best you can do.

CHAPTER 31

Handling Sexual Attraction

It's Gonna Happen

I've had a crush on many clients over the years. No, I've never had an affair, nor was I physically inappropriate. But have I had fantasies about some of my clients? Have I looked forward to seeing some of them more than they looked forward to seeing me? Have there been clients for whom there is palpable sexual chemistry, where some sessions feel more like dates and less like . . . therapy? Sure.

This will happen; it comes too easily as part of the job. After all, you're dealing with people, not filling in potholes on a residential street. Sexual chemistry and attraction come with the territory. In the literature, we talk about clients' "sexual transference." It's usually described as a common stage of therapy, especially in the beginning when clients put you on a pedestal and see you all too easily as the perfect partner, one who listens, empathizes, and offers support and kindness in their world, which is often unkind.

But there is also your side of the equation. Because of the simple intimacy of the therapy process, the potential for seduction is high. Often clients tell you things they have never said to anyone else—about their childhood abuse or struggles with addiction or thoughts that keep them on edge or awake night after night. It's hard not only to feel compassion, but also to feel . . . special and needed. Powerful stuff. And that pulls you in.

Good to know, but what do you do about it?

Your first line of defense is obviously to be aware of what is unfolding: that you are attracted and need to be careful, rather than pretending it's not happening. Then, step back and ask yourself, why this person, why now? Beyond the initial attraction, what are the relationship and your fantasies telling you about you? Is something missing in your life—that you are lonely or trying to recover from a breakup? Are you actively struggling with your own intimate relationship, and the client sitting across from you is offering what you need most—to be appreciated, feel needed, and feel important? Rather than making your relationship with your client a solution to a personal problem, think of it as a red flag letting you know that there are issues you need to work on. Next, be professional. Don't have this client be your last appointment at 7:00 P.M., if possible, because it will easily feel like a date. Don't rationalize talking about how you too have struggled in your relationship because your common problems will quickly turn into an emotional glue.

And finally, talk to your supervisor. Because secrecy fuels the excitement of affairs, you don't want to keep this attraction to yourself. No, you don't need to spill your guts to your boss about your marriage and how you haven't had sex for six months, but you can talk about how you feel in the sessions, how you feel pulled. By putting this issue on the table, you can get the support and advice you need to get it off that table. Depending on her clinical base, your supervisor may recommend transferring the client, setting firm boundaries, or talking directly about what is unfolding. Ideally, she can empathize and help you see that sexual attraction is common, that there are ways to get out of your emotional brain and into your rational, professional one.

Developing erotic feelings for your clients is one of the challenges of doing this work. It happens. Just don't let it derail you.

CHAPTER 32

Those You Can't Help

John fell into cocaine addiction, and it took its toll. He lost his marriage, his job, and his house. When I first met him, he had gradually pulled himself together—got clean, worked as a handyman in his community, and found and lived with a caring woman and her young son. But then John felt restless and wanted to return to his old life—living in Florida, doing insurance assessments, and specializing in disasters. He found a job and a great apartment in a good neighborhood where he could bike to work. But two weeks after moving, John found a way to track down cocaine and overdosed.

Sam had been married for 40 years. His wife passed away, and he was struggling. His doctor suggested that Sam talk to someone about his grief. And so he did. He came to his first session carrying photo albums of his wife, letters he had written when they were courting. We looked at the pictures, he read the letters aloud, and we talked about grief and how it unravels over time. I suggested that Sam consider medication, and he did. Within a few weeks, he felt better, reached out to his extended family, started going to church. Yes, he still had periods of sadness, but he thought he had climbed out of his gloom. We ended therapy but left the door open so that Sam could return anytime. Two years later, I received a call from his daughter; Sam had committed suicide. She wanted to talk with me. Because of confidentiality, I could say nothing, but being the executor of his estate, she had legal access to medical information. She sent me a copy of her executorship; we talked on the phone. Sam had pulled away but said things were fine. In hindsight, his daughter believed that he had gone off his medication and suspected that he was probably drinking heavily. "How did you get my name?" I asked. She replied, "We found your business card by his body."

Annie struggled with anorexia for fifteen years. She had seven admissions to treatment centers, multiple surgeries for physical problems related to the anorexia, and was at death's door several times. It was painful to watch and difficult to see history repeat itself, a struggle to not slip like her into resignation. Annie had a ton of insights, a-ha moments that lasted for a few days or weeks and then evaporated. But you never saw your efforts with her take hold. And yet somehow, she was able to finally turn it around. After so many years of struggling, Annie managed to gain momentum, began to apply the skills she had learned; her life was finally working for her, moving her toward healing in a way I never imagined. Was it her last surgery, maybe seeing younger versions of herself in a treatment that startled her into seeing herself in a new way? Yes, maybe; who knows?

When starting out as a therapist, you are undoubtedly filled with optimism; that's how it should be. But as you gain experience, you are just as undoubtedly going to meet clients for whom you see possibilities and hope, but they do not; where you know that they can make it if they just try a bit harder and follow through on your suggestions—turn that corner and not quit that job, not contact their dealer, confront their ex, get off their couch despite how they feel. They seem to gain traction, then get stuck. They try again, but then stop. You root for them louder and more consistently than anyone in their lives, continue to see potential when friends and family, for good reasons, burned out and gave up long ago. For these clients doing therapy and trying your best can feel discouraging, a continual trudge through psychological mud.

The painful downside of our profession is that you're continually dealing with the dark side of life in its myriad forms. And for some people, it is exceptionally dark: the suicides, the depression, and hopelessness that never lifts; children who will likely never shake the trauma they unfairly inherited. Not unlike emergency room docs, you do your best and sometimes find that your best just isn't good enough.

Here it's easy to blame yourself, believe that it's about your lack of skills—that someone more experienced would have seen what you didn't notice or even said what you said but said it differently, offered that perfect sentence that suddenly enabled your clients to think about themselves and their lives in a new way.

Or you think it isn't about skills but effort—that you gave up, somehow slipped into their world of depression or exhaustion where nothing matters, nothing changes. They're exhausted, and you are too; you begin to coast, feel resigned to what is. You feel guilty, but the undertow is strong, too strong. Or you don't mentally quit, but you became frustrated, and you worry that your frustration shows, and you now fear that you've gotten hooked—you're pushing them the same as everyone else in their lives. All these thoughts are normal and understandable.

This is perhaps a clinical challenge, but more often, it is an existential one, your answer to why bad things happen to good people or to people at all. Why do people like John and Sam give up on their lives, while Annie perseveres long enough to change and thrive? Because we are dealing with life so intimately, tracking so closely how people are navigating their journeys, these issues are always running in the background of the work we do.

To survive in this complicated world of relationships, problems, and pain, it helps to come up with a way of thinking about what you do that, for you, makes sense, a philosophy that is something more than a one-liner. You need a mindset and working premise that you believe in your heart as well as your mind and that can help you from slipping into cynicism and burnout.

The starting point is stepping back and defining your way of explaining your job and its limits. Think about and develop your own explanation of why some people can't turn their lives around despite all the support they receive. Come up with something, although it may change over time, about your role in people's lives and about the power or impotence of therapy and why what you do might not work.

My philosophy has been realizing that the only power I have is what I say and do when I'm talking with my client in a room for a set amount of time; acknowledging that, yes, I have some tools that can help shape people's lives, but I can't live their lives. Despite what I think about my impact and importance, I recognize that what I offer, in contrast to all that is going on in their lives, is often merely a drop in the bucket. And some days, it feels like what we have to offer seems like primitive medicine, that we're not much farther along in our skill and knowledge than those early physicians who did bloodletting and blistering.

I also believe that life is ultimately healing—you keep encountering problems, so you learn the lessons from those problems. Although Annie eventually was able to learn the moral of the story of her years, John, Sam, and many others didn't. Maybe they got lost or just ran out of time. They died or dissolved into their problems because they didn't have enough time or energy to push forward. It's sad, but maybe this is life. Maybe in the next lifetime, they will turn that corner.

The challenge here is to make some sense of your world and move on despite setbacks, to allow yourself to feel your sadness and shock, to realize that this sadness and shock are a measure of how much you care, and that caring is the true measure of who you are.

What is your philosophy? Why the pain, the suffering? What are the limits of what you can do, the limits of what is the best you can do? What can you, maybe and only maybe, do differently? Decide what you think.

PART III

YOUR WORKPLACE

Your workplace is where you live a sizeable portion of your day and week. It's a place, but it's also a community, a family of sorts that brings with it all the pluses and minuses of any family. Here we explore this new family.

CHAPTER 33

So, You Don't Like Your Supervisor?

Your impression of your supervisor during your job interview was that she was (1) okay, neutral, no red flags; (2) positive—she seemed supportive and highlighted your strengths, always a good sign; (3) extremely positive—you felt a warm connection right away; she reminded you of your grandmother; (4) other—you didn't get a chance to meet her; you did meet her, but it was a quick handshake; you were so anxious in the interview that you probably couldn't identify her in a police lineup.

But now the rubber hits the road, and you're meeting with her weekly. Something's changed; this isn't going the way you expected. She seems to harp on paperwork rather than on cases, or she asks "therapeutic questions" like "And this reminds you of whom?" Or she seems distracted in the meeting or is frankly unreliable—canceling your supervisory sessions at the last minute or not responding to emails. This relationship is not what you envisioned or need.

You can think of the supervisory relationship as an arranged marriage between professionals, but with the added bonus of a power imbalance where you're in a one-down position. While these relationships can often work out well, it's also not surprising that one of the primary reasons people quit their jobs isn't the salary or type of work, but poor rapport with their supervisors. Even a lousy job can be made better when you like and feel supported by the people around you, especially the person overseeing your work.

If you're getting off to a rocky start with your supervisor, you may think the reason is just about not knowing each other, and you need to build trust, not unlike what you have to do with clients. As with new clients, you just need to be patient, adapt, try harder, and hope things will turn around with your good efforts and attitude. That approach may work. But just in case it doesn't, here are a few suggestions to consider and try out.

Decide What's You

The director of the agency that hired me after I finished graduate school was a friendly, neutral, hands-off guy. I had little to no contact with him; he seemed to rarely be in the office, and instead was occupied with state and local coordination and committees. But just as I completed my first year on the job, he left. His replacement was a retired army colonel who had no experience in mental health and was hired primarily for his organizational and financial savvy. I was intimidated before the guy even hit the front door.

The colonel reminded me of my critical dad and, like him and unlike his predecessor, was a big presence, very much in charge, always looking over everyone's shoulders. Adding fuel to my angst was my experience in the military with drill sergeants and officers. I froze in his presence, felt like a ten-year-old, and adopted a hypervigilant, walking-on-eggshells stance. Looking back now, I couldn't shake my impressions of him and feel like the adult I was around him because I never was able to push through my assumptions and stereotypes.

My experience of this new director was about me and my little-kid triggers, and it may be part of your side of the supervisory equation as well. The way your supervisor clears her throat reminds you a bit of your critical grandmother. Or her way of reviewing your paperwork reminds you of your dad's "white-glove" inspections of your room on Saturday mornings. Maybe her lack of praise reminds you of the Eeyore-like guy you dated in college. You're seeing her through your lens of past relationships and hurtful feelings that have left you sensitive in particular ways. Your challenge is to take responsibility for yourself and the ways your own bias is interfering in the relationship.

Realize She Has Her Own Issues

Like you, your supervisor has probably got her own stuff—despite her efforts to be unbiased and professional, you still remind her of her struggling and frustrating son. Or she's struggling with personal issues—she's going through a divorce, her mother has Stage IV cancer. She doesn't respond to your emails quickly because she has to schlep her mom to chemo three days a week. Or she's harping on paperwork because her supervisor is breathing down her neck about the upcoming audit, making that paperwork a big deal.

Be Concrete about Your Problems and Needs

Not having the supervisory relationship you anticipated doesn't mean you have to take what you get. Because you're not ten years old, you need to do what you likely couldn't do with your critical grandmother, your father, or even that college date, namely, be assertive. As we discussed previously, one part of effective assertiveness is being concrete and clear about what you need. If you come to supervisory sessions with vague complaints, your supervisor will feel frustrated that she needs to do a lot of the heavy lifting to understand what you need. If this happens session after session, it can all too quickly sound like too much whining; you become that high-maintenance employee that most supervisors don't appreciate.

So help her out. Be clear about what you need help with: that you need tips on managing a particular clinical problem, on how to coordinate with another agency, or specific training in using the software or filling out forms, or doing play therapy. If you're clear, she'll likely be more helpful, and you both can leave meetings feeling satisfied.

Follow Her Expectations

She wants you to have a clear agenda and send it to her ahead of your meeting; she needs a quick rundown of your caseload every other week; she's big on promptness and expects the paperwork in by 4:00 on Friday and no later. What if none of these expectations suits your style? Too bad. She is your boss and has a right to set expectations.

Don't think of her demands as being about power or about being forced to conform to her rules, but as a process of building a relationship of trust. Clients begin to trust you when you don't double-book their sessions, when you are focused during their sessions, and when you sensitively respond to their concerns. By your doing what you need to do, they come to feel safe. Similarly, you learn to trust your clients when they pay their bills, give sufficient notice about canceling, and do the homework you suggest; you see them taking you and therapy seriously.

It is much the same for you and your supervisor. You want her to be available when she says she will be available and to answer your questions without any critical attitude. For her, it's about your showing up on time and having an agenda prepared. You build trust in relationships by clarifying what you need most and then seeing if the other person can deliver.

Focus on yourself. Do your part; see what happens next.

Fine-Tune the Relationship

Eventually you may find that she lapses into long clinical lectures that you have difficulty following, or that she sporadically cancels supervisory sessions that leave you feeling annoyed and clinically adrift. As in any relationship, problems naturally arise, and the challenge is to address them rather than sweep them under the rug.

A good supervisor will initiate this problem solving and fine-tuning early on by asking, "How are we doing?" This is your opportunity to speak up. If this question catches you off guard and you don't do well thinking on your feet, punt—"Thanks for asking; can I think about it and we can talk about it next time?" But if she doesn't ask and you're not getting what you need, it's time for you to speak up.

Again, focus on what you need rather than complaining about what you're not getting. Just as you frame your concerns with your clients in terms of their presenting problems ("Because you are so worried about John's school performance, I think an evaluation for ADHD may be helpful"), frame your needs in terms of her concerns: "The paperwork software seems confusing, and it takes me a long time to complete it, creating these delays," "I'm wondering if we can do quick check-ins about my clients a couple of times a week, rather than feeling rushed during our supervisory meetings," or "Can I send you an email with the status of my caseload to save time in our supervisory session?" Unless clients speak up, it's too easy for you to assume that everything is fine. The same can happen between you and your supervisor.

Ask about a Transfer

Okay, you feel you've done your best to sort out what's you and what's her and to be clear and reliable, but nothing has changed. You have reached a point where you think you both are simply not compatible.

If you have exhausted your strategies, the problem is ultimately back in your lap. Solve your problem. Find out if you can transfer to another supervisor or another team. The answer is probably no, especially in a small agency, but ask anyway. Then, decide what other options you have and what you want to do next: transfer to a different section if it is a large agency or talk to human resources about options to resolve the problem. If you don't see any options for improving your work environment within your organization, start looking for another job.

This is the worst-case scenario, and rarely does it come to this, but your job is at least one-third of your everyday life. You are not an indentured servant, and you need to decide what is the best use of your time. Be proactive. Don't be a victim of a bad work environment.

CHAPTER 34

What Your Supervisor's World Is Like

Your supervisor's got the easiest job in the world. She sits in her office doing who knows what while you see back-to-back clients with only a quick lunch break. Or she's not even in her office; she's off to some in-house meeting where she chats with other supervisors or to a three-day state conference where they probably quit at 4:00 and do happy hour, while you still have a couple more clients to see.

You're right: your supervisor probably does some or all of those things. I used to have the same thoughts about my supervisors, off somewhere or tucked away in their cozy offices shuffling papers, writing out their shopping lists for the weekend—ho-hum—until I or a few other staff members came in for weekly meetings. But then I became a supervisor, and boy was I in shock. I'd hit my desk at 8:00 on a Monday morning and find there were 300 emails in my in-box. My boss would have left an urgent message about the budget—revenue's down 50K for the month, and we needed to talk. And as I walked down the hall to go to the bathroom, three or four staff people were not saying good morning but waving their hands in varying degrees of desperation or stopping me to ask if they could ask me a quick question (it's never a quick question) sometime that morning.

A supervisor's work life is usually filled with more reaction than action, maybe even more so than the lives of the clinicians they oversee. Supervisors operate in the gray zone of middle management, the sandwich generation of any agency with directors and CEOs above and line staff below, and so have to serve two masters. The administrators above focus on budget, public perceptions, and ornery board members who really don't understand the agency. The staff below are struggling with caseloads, stupid paperwork, and crises generated by clients in forever emotional turmoil. The supervisor has to walk between these different worlds. She is a translator—trying to explain to the folks above why big caseloads or stupid paperwork does impact the budget or the community's perceptions, while trying to explain to the staff why the stupid paperwork isn't stupid but clinically sound, and that the caseload swells are temporary or are opportunities to be creative in our clinical approaches so we can provide the greatest mental health good for the greatest number.

I know, you're not particularly feeling sorry for her—that's why she gets the big bucks and why she still has the cozy office. You're right. But your initial impression of what she does all day may be wrong. She is hardly slouching, doing crossword puzzles and texting with her son about his new puppy. What she likely is doing is:

- Sorting through those hundreds of emails, mostly garbage, about changes in state regulations, about surveys that some government agency needs to be completed by this Thursday, about mandatory training on hand-washing procedures that all staff need to complete and have entered into their personnel record by the end of next week.
- Fielding a call from human resources that the number-one candidate for the open clinical position didn't pass the background check or drug screening and has been eliminated. Now she needs to readvertise and start over, which worries her about caseloads, revenue, and so on.
- Needing to go to the annual three-day meeting on legislation updates impacting the agency. She's assigned to a workgroup looking at PR to influence state legislators on upcoming mental health bills, including working dinners and long nights and trips to the state capital to lobby. The most boring activities in the world, and she hasn't found anyone yet who can check in on her 80-year-old mother.
- Fine-tuning an updated Excel spreadsheet on revenue projections for the next quarter that is due Friday, but the financial folks haven't found the latest figures for some reason, and she sucks at using Excel.
- Needing to talk with Ani about the status of her suicidal client to determine whether he needs inpatient care. This is the stuff that can keep her awake at 3:00 A.M. Oh, she probably needs to talk

with Rob about his paperwork—his progress notes are behind—and to speak with HR about whether his lateness qualifies for a Category One offense.

- Worrying that her boss doesn't quite understand how the large caseloads are impacting revenue and staff retention, and that he won't adequately explain it when he makes his monthly report to the board. She needs to crunch numbers to show how much training new staff costs and send it to him by Friday.
- Starting to set up that staffwide training on autism as a stepping-stone to initiating a new clinical program specifically for children on the spectrum. While she's at it, she needs to consider applying for an NIH grant.
- Needing to ask if John, her more experienced clinician, can set up group supervision for the interns arriving in two months. She also needs to ask him if he would be willing to represent the agency on the interagency committee investigating mental health services for the homeless.
- Needing to remember to ask Kate to do a self-evaluation to prepare for her upcoming probationary evaluation.

You get the idea. Do you feel sorry for her? Don't. Just recognize her world isn't quite as cozy as you may think.

CHAPTER 35

Time to Leave Your Therapist?

When I meet couples, I regularly ask if either or both of them are in individual therapy. Fairly often, at least one partner will say yes.

"And how long have you been in therapy?"

"Awhile. Think I've been seeing Sarah for a few years."

"And what are you working on with her?"

"Oh, anxiety and stuff."

Twenty minutes into the session, when the same client is talking about his uncontrolled anxiety and demonstrating it on the spot, I wonder (although I know I just met the person and don't have any baseline) how much of that anxiety-and-stuff therapy is really working.

Now I have nothing against Sarah. But the thought lurking beneath my furrowed brow is that sometimes therapy, for a lot of good reasons, simply isn't doing what it's supposed to. Yet both the client and the therapist plod along together seemingly forever. What's going on? Is this some blink contest, a case of the emperor's new clothes, a failure to talk about the elephant in the room, or something else?

I'm especially concerned about the client who has never been in therapy before. Unlike veterans who have learned what works and what doesn't for them through trial and error, these therapy newbies lack this knowledge. Because they don't know what to expect, because of the power difference, and because they are struggling and often have limited options, it's easy for them to take what they get, to become the passive consumer who assumes the doctor knows best.

It is vital to the success of therapy that the client trust the therapist's judgment. Just the same, it is vital that both the client and the therapist question whether what they're doing is really working.

To help you grapple with that question, I'd like to propose a thought experiment: If you were to write a brochure that your agency would place in its waiting room about client rights, empowerment, and quality assurance, what would you say? Here's mine; see what you think.

Is It Time to Stop Therapy or Find Someone New?

Thank you for trusting us with your mental health services. Maybe you've been in therapy before, or this is your first experience; perhaps you've been seeing your therapist for weeks, months, or longer. Maybe you found those first few sessions especially helpful—just having someone to listen and talk to relieved a lot of your anxiety. But now that things have settled down, maybe you're wondering if this isn't quite as good a fit as you initially thought. It could be that your personalities seem to clash, or your therapist's approach and style aren't what you think you need for the longer haul. You may be thinking of terminating. Or maybe you feel like the sessions lately have been dragging—that your therapist doesn't have much to say, you both seem to cover the same ground each week, or you don't feel your initial concerns have improved that much. But at the same time, the idea of starting over with someone else feels overwhelming or a bit depressing.

A therapeutic relationship is probably different from the other relationships in your life, but it's still a relationship. And, like any relationship, it's helpful to periodically step back and see how well it is or is not working, to pay attention to your reactions and feelings. We realize that evaluating a relationship can be hard to do: You might not be sure if you should trust these feelings, you think you maybe just need to give it more time, or that as you do with your doctor, you're looking to your therapist to be the one in charge who knows best.

Here are some questions and suggestions to ask yourself that may help you decide what to do:

DO YOU FEEL SAFE?

Therapy is often about discussing things that are hard for you to talk about and to take that risk you need to feel safe—not worry about being judged, criticized, or dismissed. While it's normal to feel anxious in the first few sessions as you get to know each other, at some point, you should begin to relax, to settle, and to not worry that you have to be careful about what you say. If the safety isn't there, you're not going to get the most out of your sessions.

DO YOU FEEL LIKE YOU ARE TREADING WATER?

Like learning any new skills and ways of thinking, repetition is part of the process—circling back to the same themes or behaviors to help you incorporate changes into your everyday life. But you should understand the connection between what you are focusing on and your presenting concerns. You should feel that you are making progress, even if slowly, rather than feeling like you are talking about problems that don't address your pressing concerns or that there's no forward movement.

If you're feeling like you're stuck at a plateau, it may be because the safety you need isn't there, and you're understandably holding back. Or it may be that you and your therapist have both fallen into a comfortable routine that isn't providing what you need. Or perhaps there actually isn't much more to talk about—the problems you originally had are largely behind you, but you enjoy the relationship with your therapist, that connection, and are reluctant to give therapy up.

Time to step back and ask yourself if your therapy is giving you what you need—helping you solve problems or providing the support right now to get through a rough patch. Or does it feel like you're treading water or have outgrown the need?

DO YOU FEEL THAT THE THERAPIST'S STYLE AND APPROACH ARE A GOOD FIT?

If you feel like you and your therapist are not a good fit—that she talks too much or too little, or that her way of thinking about problems just seems foreign and unhelpful to you—you want to pay attention to these gut reactions. Ask yourself: Do you generally feel better when you walk out than when you walked in? Do you feel your therapist understands you, and do you understand what she is doing and why?

WHAT MIGHT BE TRIGGERING YOUR REACTIONS? HAVE YOU BEEN HERE BEFORE?

If the answer to the second question is yes, you might examine why. Does what you're feeling in therapy seem familiar? Have you had similar reactions or problems in other relationships—that you perhaps are sensitive to being judged and so hold back; or you linger although you've outgrown the relationship; or if you're feeling pressed to deal with issues outside your comfort zone, you become anxious, find yourself thinking this isn't working, and want to leave? This recreation of patterns often occurs in the therapy process, and while it's your therapist's job to help you recognize and possibly change these old ways of coping, it may be helpful for you to do the same.

TIME TO SPEAK UP

If you feel your therapy isn't meeting your expectations, we'd like to encourage you to discuss your feelings with your therapist. If initiating this conversation within a session seems too overwhelming, send your therapist an email laying out your questions and concerns and then follow up with a face-to-face conversation. You can also prompt your therapist to take the lead: Say at the end of a session that you'd like to take some time in the next session to get your therapist's feedback about goals, progress, and next steps. This heads-up will give you both time to step back, take stock, and help jump-start the conversation.

Ideally, the result of that conversation is a clear plan for moving forward: that your therapist understands what you need to feel safe or how to shift the focus so that you are no longer treading water. If you both agree that you have possibly outgrown the need for therapy, you might decide to take a break or to try spreading out sessions and see how you feel. And if you realize that working with this therapist simply is not a good fit, you have agreed on what's needed for a smooth transition or amicable termination.

Our practice and administration are here to support you in any way we can. Our goal is to help you achieve your goals. Feel free to let us know how we can help.

So what do you think about my brochure? Agree, disagree? Anything you would want to change, include, or drop?

If you agree with most of these ideas, realize that you've just given yourself a challenge: You need to work your side of the relationship equation and ask yourself the same questions: What do you need to do to help clients feel safe? Can you recognize when you are running on routines or treading water because you enjoy the relationship and don't want to let it go, or because you've reached the limits of your skills and erroneously believe that more of the same will eventually provide the cure? Are you comfortable taking the pulse of the relationship periodically to ensure that you and your client are on the same page? Just as clients need to take stock of the relationship and think about the progress they've made, so do you.

Grappling with this stuff will be good for your clients and good for you as a professional. If you feel you're struggling with any of these issues, don't hesitate to talk to your supervisor or a trusted colleague and get the advice and support you need.

CHAPTER 36

Clients Are Not Vicarious Outlets

Jackie is considering divorce. Her partner sounds like an ogre—controlling, manipulative, self-centered, and even, at times, emotionally abusive. She's fed up, and you can understand why. You find yourself supporting her decision, that yes, she has a right to stand up for herself, push back or get out and simply not take what she gets. It's not about divorce, you say, but empowerment.

Good strategy? Sure, but you may need to be careful. If you are having trouble in your own intimate relationship, are feeling controlled, say, by your supervisor, or struggle with conflict and avoid confrontation, the danger here is that Jackie becomes a vicarious outlet for your "stuff."

Here's where we get into countertransference, projection, overidentification, and other assorted emotional dangers that the mechanic at the garage or the billing person at the water department likely never worries about. Blurring the line between your stuff and someone else's stuff is often part of our even casual relationships, where we see others through our lenses, compare them to ourselves, feel their anxiety, and heap on advice. But all this emotional investment is magnified in therapy because you and I are in positions of influence, and that power combined with our humanity can be dangerous.

Be careful not to use clients to do what you cannot. You encourage Jackie to stand up to her husband or explore divorce not only because she needs to be proactive in her life but because, at least in part, you need to do so as well. Or you discover that she has unresolved grief from a childhood loss, which resonates with your unresolved loss—and reinforces your argument for her need to take time to explore that past (because you are essentially using the work with her as a vicarious outlet for your healing). Or perhaps worst of all, you step into being the supportive partner that Jackie doesn't have for one hour a week. She doesn't divorce her partner or change and stand up to him, but instead leans on you to help her cope. She becomes dependent on you, but you also become dependent on her for the intimacy or appreciation you lack in your own life.

How can you avoid having clients become vicarious outlets?

Know Your Vulnerabilities

If you do have lingering grief from your past, recognize that that wound can be easily activated, causing you either to be overly focused on these issues with clients or to quickly minimize them. Similarly, if you have a history of abuse, you can overidentify with Jackie or the six-year-old child suffering from abuse as well.

Know Your Response

Your issues make clients' problems stand out, and so you push clients to deal with them before they are willing or ready to do so. Or you take the opposite stance—minimize and avoid—for example, telling parents concerned about their son's pot use that it is part of the teen's normal experimentation as you recall your own adolescent (or current) pot use.

Know Your Immediate Stressors

If you are going through a rough patch in your own intimate relationships, acknowledge that Jackie and her issues will be triggers that can distort and bias your view and strategy. If you're struggling with your own dependency on marijuana or with your supervisor who seems controlling, make sure you start therapy with a clear eye and focus. Better yet, if a client's issues spark intrusive thoughts or emotions in you, talk about transferring the case.

Look for Themes

"You teach best what you need to learn most." It's not just Jackie who you're encouraging to step up and empower, but most of your clients. You may rationalize that your clinical model drives your consistent focus on developing assertiveness in clients, and it may be, but the investment, the pushing, the across-the-board emotional intensity you notice in your behavior with clients tell you it is not just your clinical stance or values motivating that focus, but your own needs.

Have Clear Models and Treatment Maps

If you lack a firm clinical foundation and are winging it because you don't really know what to do with specific clients or problems, your emotions and triggers will take over.

Get Consultation

Talk to your supervisor or a trusted experienced colleague about the need for a clinical frame to lean on, about the skills you need to stay in your rational brain and out of your emotional one. Talk about the patterns and themes you see—about your vulnerability working with folks like Jackie—so they can help you separate yourself from your clients and provide you with the clear-eyed support you need to stay on track.

Solve Your Problems

Get couple therapy, talk to your supervisor about your relationship with her, and get individual therapy to put past wounds to rest.

Take a few minutes, every now and then, and check in with yourself. What are your vulnerabilities? How do you respond when triggered? What support, advice, or training do you need to circumvent these dangers? What do you need to do to put your problems to rest?

CHAPTER 37

When You Don't Like Your Clients

You're frustrated: Jim never comes to his sessions with an agenda and never does the homework he agreed to, although he has a million reasons why. You're irritated and annoyed with Mary: She keeps repeating the same complaints and stories over and over; despite your best efforts to change the course of the session, you feel like you are both treading water. And there's Charles, who seems to go in and out of crisis—nothing much to talk about one week, but is calling you four times a day the next. You're never sure whether Charles will show up; you see his phone number and dread picking up the phone. Finally, there's five-year-old Brett, who has encopresis; appointments with him and his parents feel like you are groping through a fog, unable to see where you're going.

If you feel this way, don't beat yourself up. Meeting and connecting with clients can feel a bit like meeting strangers at a cocktail party: You quickly join with Jack and look forward to seeing him; Simone, not so much, but it's fine because the therapy is going well. But then there are others—the Jims, Marys, Charleses, and Bretts. These are the clients whose sessions you brace yourself for; you look at tomorrow's schedule, sigh, and say to yourself, "It's okay, I can get through this."

Face it: you can't like all your clients. At the cocktail party you could say, "It was good to meet you," walk away, and never have to worry about seeing that person again. But at work you probably don't have much control over your caseload. Consider that not liking clients, or dreading seeing them, is often a symptom of other issues at work. Here are a few to consider.

You're Doing the Heavy Lifting

At first, you thought Jim's passive, not-follow-through stance was linked to his anxiety about therapy. But lately, you wonder if this is just Jim—you've had hints that his agreeable-but-no-follow-through style has been much the same with his boss, his partner, and his past relationships. When you're washing dishes or mowing the lawn, you find yourself wondering how to help Jim be more proactive.

You're working harder than Jim.

What to Do

While your instincts may be to try harder to find that magic bullet that will turn Jim around, the starting point is assessing the situation. Specifically, despite seeming to want therapy, Jim isn't doing therapy. He doesn't have much to say, and he doesn't have an agenda. He says he wants help to change, but he isn't doing the homework. You're like the family doctor who gives him a prescription that he tosses into the trash the moment he walks out the door. You need to uncover the problem under the problem. It's not about content (no need to plod through his latest reason for not doing his homework) but the process: that you and Jim seem to be out of step, that the problem you think you're working on may not be the one he wants helps with, that your approach is not what he was expecting. And yes, it's okay to say that you feel you're working harder than he is. Put his problems back in his lap.

Countertransference

As you work with Mary, you find yourself feeling irritated. As you did with Jim, you need to address the treading of water, the possible being out of step. But your growing irritation is likely about you. Maybe Mary reminds you of your father, who constantly repeated the same things over and over, or your partner, who keeps falling into the same conversational rut. Or actually, Mary looks a bit like your ex and has that same way of pointing her finger at you when she is getting ramped up and wants to argue.

What to Do

Know your vulnerable points. Maybe people like Mary remind you of your father or your ex, or perhaps you are particularly sensitive to aggressive women or passive men. Gaining this awareness is half the battle. The other half is learning to catch your reactions when they are triggered and being able to prevent them from distorting the clinical relationship. This is a time to talk to your supervisor about circumventing these situations in straightforward behavioral ways. Better yet, consider a stint of therapy to help you separate the past from the present.

High Maintenance

Charles seems to go from crisis to crisis. Unlike with Jim, you're not working harder than he is; unlike Mary, you're not being emotionally triggered. You're just worn out, tired of being on a perpetual roller coaster.

What to Do

These clients are difficult. They may have personality disorders. Frequently they have histories laden with trauma. Here you need support and guidance from your supervisor, a clear diagnosis and plan, and often a team of others—a psychiatrist, a family-support person, a peer counselor—who are on board and are able to support you so you can go off duty at times.

You're Over Your Head

For a client like Brett, you need specific clinical skills. Because you're likely more a generalist than a specialist and can't pick and choose your caseload, you will invariably have clients you have no treatment map for or little experience working with. You're fumbling about in some play-therapy way. You're doing a lot of faking-it-till-you-make-it, and there's a lot of faking it going on.

What to Do

What you're already doing isn't an option. For good reasons, you're really not doing your job of providing quality treatment. Your other two options are get the training and the session-by-session coaching you need to get you out of the fog or let your supervisor know that you're not yet ready to take on Brett and that he would be better served by someone more experienced.

Your connection with clients is on a continuum. For those you struggle with, step back and look beyond the surface for patterns and underlying problems and then get the information and assistance you need to deal with them.

And most of all, don't give yourself a hard time. That you don't like some clients will always be part of your work long term. What you want to figure out now is what is you, what is them, and what you need to do to move forward.

CHAPTER 38

Working in Challenging Environments

You love your office chair and the way your office is decorated, so that it's comfy for you and your clients. And when you're in a session, there are no interruptions; once the door is closed, it's quiet, allowing you and your client to settle. But sometimes you're not in your work cocoon because you work in a different setting—a home, a hospital, or a school. Or you're doing teletherapy, living in the online universe. Each environment creates its own challenges and opportunities.

Homes

Working in a client's home is tough. You often have appointments in the late afternoon or evening in parts of town where you've never been. There's a scary pit bull on the porch or three flights of dimly lit stairs to navigate. And once you get inside, you're likely greeted by more pets, little kids happy to see you, someone cooking in the kitchen, grandpa yelling from the back bedroom, cigarette smoke filling the air, ambient noise from a television somewhere. You're out of your comfort zone; this isn't your comfy office.

Home visits pose the biggest challenges. Not only is the home the client's environment, not yours, but there's so much going on, so much stimulation that you can't control. There is no closing of the consulting room door and silence. Instead, there's chaos and distraction—the dinner burning on the stove, a neighbor knocking on the door, the teenager refusing to come out of her room, grandpa still yelling. And then the dog wanders in, and it takes ten minutes to get him to settle down and stay put. Your first therapeutic goal is often just getting everyone together in the same room, sitting still.

On the upside, home visits make therapy more convenient for clients. By meeting with you at 6:00 P.M. instead of needing to come to your office at 4:00, they don't have to lose time from work, which removes an obstacle to following through. Since home is where they live, you also can gain a fuller picture of the clients' world and their routines. You get to meet grandpa (if you can get him out of the back bedroom), who would never be able to come to your office; you see the level of poverty and chaos; and you see the family's caring for each other. And if you're able to create some intimacy or privacy, clients often are more open and relaxed; there's no performance pressure they can feel when sitting in your office; multitasking becomes an asset—mom opens up about her struggles during the week while cooking the chicken in her own kitchen. The six-year-old fiddles with her doll as she talks about the bully at school.

How do you work in such a setting? You don't want simply to take what you get, be the passenger on the train. Decide what you need to do your job. Take time in the first session to create some agreed-upon rules of engagement—that the family will meet all together in the living room, or that you will meet with the primary client on the back porch where there is more privacy, or that you will both go for a walk around the block. Negotiate rules about no phones, or put a sign on the door to notify the door-knocking neighbor. Crucially, have the head of household rather than you be the enforcer of the rules, so there is ownership of and buy-in to the process. Let the family know that you want them to have an agenda, so you're not sitting in silence just long enough for some distraction to take over and disrupt the process.

Also confirm the home visit beforehand. In my experience, clients or families tend to forget you're coming. Going out to make an appointment—to your office or to the family doctor—is psychologically different from having the appointment come to you. At home, it's easy for clients to get caught up in their lives, lose track of time, run out to the grocery store, and not get back in time. It's also easier for clients who are ambivalent or resistant about therapy to find reasons not to be there or to use distractions to avoid serious conversations. If using distraction or not showing up becomes a pattern, you want to address it to uncover the emotional problem under the problem.

Finally, consider your own safety. Unlike working in your office, working in a client's home gives you less control and support. Family members may be drinking, or there may be guns in the house. Almost all agencies have a system for the staff to let their supervisor or team know what home they are going to and when they are going. Use it. If you have any safety concerns, bring them up with your supervisor and the family. Some ways to address such concerns include going out in pairs or doing home visits only in daylight hours, refusing to visit when a boyfriend is there, or even not permitting home visits. It's your responsibility to speak up and ultimately protect yourself.

Schools

As in a client's home, there are advantages and disadvantages of working in a school rather than in your office. You can see your clients in their world—in the halls, the classroom, and the playground. Clients may be more relaxed. You can often easily pull in friends who can be a support or source of information; catch a teacher, guidance counselor, or principal to compare notes and get updates; or more easily set up a student–teacher–you meeting during lunch break.

If you're sitting in on a one-time or periodic special event—supporting parents in a quarterly teacher–parent conference, consulting with a guidance counselor about a student, attending a quarterly status meeting—the school staff are prepared and will stage the meeting. But if you are meeting with a student or a group of students as a member of the school staff or meeting with them as an outside resource person, there can be distractions and situations you can't control—the fire drill, the bell ringing for the next period. Your client has difficulty focusing because she is too worried about her next-period math exam and would prefer to be cramming rather than talking to you.

As you need to do with home-based clients, you want to have clear expectations and rules of engagement. Make sure you have the privacy you need, even if it's backstage in the auditorium or on the empty playground, rather than being squeezed into a corner of the science lab where the teacher is coming in and out. If you are coming in as an outside resource, make sure you have the support from the principal and the staff for your being there. Without clarity about what you are doing and their backing, it's easy for the staff to view you as more an interruption in their work rather than as a team member.

Finally, if you are working as an outside resource, know who needs to know, the chain of command. I've supervised graduate students and staff members who go to work in a school with a particular student or a group of students who are behaviorally struggling or feel bullied. If they are concerned about a student—if Sara, for example, has suicidal ideation—who needs to be informed—me as the supervisor, the principal, the contact at the graduate school? Who is the point person for notifying parents? Who is responsible for what can get confusing fast. You or your supervisor need to have clear protocols in advance so you don't have to scramble when a crisis arises.

Hospitals

All of these challenges and needs equally apply when working in a hospital. As in the home and at school, there will undoubtedly be distractions. Maybe your patient is in a shared room; there will be interruptions for medical reasons—checking monitors, setting up IVs. You'll need to be clear about your needs—having a quiet space to talk to the family about discharge planning or scheduling a meeting with your bed-bound patient when her roommate is out for physical therapy. Like the colleagues you work with in schools, if you give the nursing staff a heads-up about what you need and what you're doing, they will try to respect your wishes or let you know what might be a better time for visits. And as in working in schools, you want to know to whom to pass on important information—nurses, doctors, or specialists like a psychiatrist.

Teletherapy

Off-site therapy has been around for a long time. In his famous case of Little Hans, Freud treated the boy through the medium of time—via letters filled with his clinical advice, which he sent to the boy's father. Our current forms of social media hit their stride with the pandemic and are here to stay. Like home-based work, teletherapy provides a way of reaching clients who might not otherwise be reached—shut-ins, folks without transportation, or folks who live too far away. It also offers potential clients a wider pool of clinicians—at least professionals in their own state and often outside of it and even in other countries. And you can even talk at the same time with couples or family members who are in different locations or use texting to get quick responses. What's not to like?

What's not to like are the current limits of the medium itself. On a screen, you often see only the heads of clients and not their entire bodies; connections can be poor—the sound goes out or off-line at a critical moment; images freeze or are dark; you can't tell if Maggie is starting to cry or not; you can't quite squeeze everyone in the frame. And there are the unwelcomed distractions—the knock on the client's door, the cat jumping on the table and blocking the screen, the baby fussing—ways, as in home-based work, that clients can disrupt the conversation and avoid. And then there is the equivalent of stomping out of the office—clients say the computer camera stopped working or that they are losing reception and need to leave the session, or they get upset and simply click you off.

Again be flexible but also assertive and agree on guidelines: That the cat stays out of the room, that they look for a location with better reception, that you schedule the appointment when the baby is likely to nap, and that you let them know you are not checking texts after 6:00 P.M. To compensate for missing some of that nonverbal information, you need to listen more intensely to pick up on changes in voice tone; you need to be more direct and ask Maggie if she is feeling upset when you can't clearly see her eyes but suspect that she is. And make sure you are working your side of the equation—that your internet connection is strong and that your space evokes comfort and intimacy, rather than being a distraction, and is not filled with your own interruptions.

Many clinicians are now doing a mix of online and office visits, which provides flexibility. Ed isn't feeling well enough to drive all the way into town for his appointment or is afraid he is contagious and doesn't want to spread his germs, but he's fine talking on his phone. Molly has to work overtime and can't make her late afternoon appointment, but she can sit in her car during lunch and have a session through her phone. Some clinicians and often many clients like the initial session to be in the office if possible so both sides can have a more complete experience. Most of the time, you may be okay with telesessions, but also be clear about your preferences—while you're comfortable doing teletherapy with teens, you're not comfortable trying to do play therapy remotely with young children; that you are willing to do check-ins with an individual, couple, or family, but if you want to do something more experiential—for example, family sculpture or teaching meditation—you'd rather wait or find a way to see clients in your office. Develop your own preferences and protocols in advance so you again don't feel you're scrambling.

The keys to working in out-of-office environments are being clear about the challenges and your needs and being creative and flexible about making it all work.

CHAPTER 39

When You're Having a Hard Time

You might not be splitting rocks with rocks, but there will be some days when the work feels hard. Although you're spending your days in a chair, and (to the outsider) simply talking, an old-fashioned, rock-breaking weariness can set in. You're tired—of people and their problems, of waking up in the middle of the night worrying if Ted might be really more depressed than he says he is, of still feeling that undertow of sadness for the child who lost his parent. You're sad that people's lives are so filled with problems that seem outside not only their control but your own as well. You're frustrated that you can't do more.

And so, you ruminate, aren't sleeping, are drinking too much, are snapping at your partner or kids every day, or are dreading work on Monday. You fantasize about being a school counselor or selling carpets with your brother-in-law. You're burned out and fed up.

It happens to all of us who do this kind of work. Partly it is the nature of the work itself: the lawyer doesn't sleep the week before a trial; the salesman is tired of hustling and being on the road; even the well-paid football player has days when his body is simply not doing what it should, and on a bad day he worries about how long he can keep this up. Will this pass? Will you bounce back? Likely.

But some people don't. Three therapists in my small community committed suicide in the past several years; psychiatrists have one of the highest suicide rates among all professions (Wang, 2019). Sure, it's sadly about them losing a battle with their own demons, but it's hard not to think that the work they did, what we do, isn't in some way part of the picture.

Just as you want to help your clients uncover what's the hard in the hardness of their lives, it helps for you to do the same. Here are some thoughts to consider when you're struggling.

You've Taken On Too Much

Your supervisor has asked if you can provide some coverage for Anne while she's on maternity leave, and your caseload has jumped. Or you've been asked to serve on a committee that reevaluates personnel policies. Or it's not about work, but you volunteered to coach your son's soccer team. You're stretched too thin, and even the weight of a feather tips the scale out of balance.

If this is temporary—the maternity leave is over in a week, the soccer season ends in a month—it's about being kind to yourself, building in as much self-care as you can—the sleeping, eating, and exercise combination that works for you. But if it's part of a bigger pattern of having a hard time saying no, as we discussed in Chapter 6, this may be about you—your personality, your "I'm happy if you're happy" stance. This is about taking the risk of being assertive, setting boundaries, and tolerating others' being unhappy with you. Talk to your supervisor about your caseload, pass on the coaching, or be an assistant coach to reduce the pressure.

Self-Criticism and Expectations

You're burning out because your anxious/critical voice is piling on. Your anxious mind tells you that if you don't want to feel that dread on Monday morning, you need to try harder to do better on your job. These are unrealistic, irrational expectations that you can never meet. Get a reality check from your supervisor about what is expected from someone at your pay grade. Take a deep breath and realize when your critical voice has taken over, pummeling you with the bad news you don't deserve. Push back.

Not Solving a Problem in Your Personal Life

You're dragging and dreading Mondays not because of the job but because the weekends lately have been a slog through hell. You've been arguing nonstop with your partner; your weekends are filled with kid soccer games and ballet lessons, and you have no time for yourself. Or your mother keeps calling wondering how you are—you realize that she is lonely, but you feel like you're doing therapy with her every weekend. The strain of it all is wearing you down.

Unlike the computer tech who probably has one brain for work and another for her personal life, your brain is not split in two—your work and personal life blend together. Staying well is about setting boundaries with your mother about her calls, stepping back and looking at your lifestyle choices, and maybe cutting back on all those games and lessons, having that heart-to-heart conversation with your partner about the arguments or starting couple therapy. Take active steps to address these issues or put them to rest. Clear out your in-box.

Know Your Stress

It's a chicken-and-egg scenario: Is your drinking too much, having a hard time saying no, or snapping at your partner a symptom of another issue or the issue itself? If these issues come and go, the question is, why today? What's the trigger? If they are more persistent, if there is a larger pattern, maybe it's time to tackle these problems head-on.

Step back and see if you can figure it out. If you need help, talk to someone—a close friend, relative, or therapist.

Life is about ups and downs, good and sour moods, doing too much or not enough. Some days your job will suck; other days, with luck, will be the best days ever. The trick is to figure out what causes the bad days and learn to fix or accept them and to build on the good ones. Learn about yourself, find that balance between your inner and outer life, live your life in a way that meets the needs of your clients and family and, more important, you. You've got time to figure this all out. Experiment. This is part of the challenge and adventure of living.

CHAPTER 40

So, What Do You Do All Day?

Working at a job usually means spending a good chunk of time in one place, and how you spend that time determines your job satisfaction. If you see six clients in a row with only a three-minute bathroom break between appointments, or if you are putting out crisis fires all day long (and you don't work in emergency services), you'll burn out quickly. On the other hand, if your day is filled with bureaucratic flotsam—filling out seemingly irrelevant forms, plowing through brain-numbing policy papers, you're likely to say, "This is not what I went to grad school for."

Generally, what works for most folks is some mix of tasks that fits your personality and working style. But what mix is the best? In his bestseller, *The 7 Habits of Highly Effective People* (2020), Stephen Covey said we can divide all work tasks into two continuums—urgent/not urgent and important/not important. Let's walk through the different combinations and as we do, think about the tasks you do in a day or week.

Urgent/Not Important

It's 9:00 on a Tuesday morning, and you get an email from human resources. HR needs you to fill in the attached spreadsheet with the names and Social Security numbers of all the clients you have seen in the last month, and it's needed by 3:00 today. Or your supervisor says in a staff meeting that the state requires that everyone complete an online training on blood-borne pathogens, and the deadline is Friday. She sighs and rolls her eyes as she says this, because she and everyone else in the room know that this training has absolutely no relevance to your work.

These kinds of tasks are the stuff that comes with working in bureaucratic settings. They are urgent because there are tight deadlines. And while they are undoubtedly crucial to HR or to the state mental health department for some reason (usually because a higher-up thinks it is essential), they are not important to you because they are not an essential part of your job. If these situations only arise occasionally, don't grumble; just do what's required. If these situations occur a lot, they are usually a symptom of poor organization, a lack of supportive infrastructure, or both.

What can you do about urgent but not important tasks at your level? You can always raise the issue in a team meeting or supervisory session, wondering aloud if there is a way for you (and your colleagues) to have more notice, so these last-minute tasks don't derail your day. Similarly, if a lack of infrastructure is the source of the problem—"Can we hire someone who can pull together these spreadsheets, or can IT develop software to capture this information automatically, so I don't have to take time away from seeing clients?" Say it, and you're done.

But if you do speak up, do it right. Speaking up is not about grousing, a poor-me complaint about how busy you are and how hard you work. That complaint will go nowhere—everyone up and down the line feels that they are busy and working hard; you're not that special snowflake. Instead, the key to voicing any complaints to your supervisor is to talk in her language by linking your concerns to what she most cares about in her world, which is usually money, community reputation, and overall quality control. So you point out to her that having to do the spreadsheet yourself forces you to reschedule three clients at the last minute, which affects how the community views the agency's services and reduces the day's revenue by 50%. You've now done the best you can do. What happens next is out of your hands.

Urgent/Important

It's 4:55 on a Friday, and you're wrapping up your session with your client Jack. He's spent the hour rambling on about the trials and tribulations of the week, and you ask how he has handled it all. He says he's been really depressed. How depressed, you ask. "Actually," he says,

"I've been feeling that I don't think I can take all this anymore, that it would be better if I just weren't here."

This is probably not a good time to look at your watch and say, "Whoa, sorry to hear. We're just about out of time. Let's pick this up next week." Instead, you're going to assess further, find out just how strong his suicidal thoughts are, whether he has a solid plan, whether you need to get him into a hospital or get an emergency custody order. Following through with him is part of your job, and it's urgent and important. This occasionally happens.

But, as with the urgent/not important tasks, if you are constantly dealing with urgent crises, you want to wonder why. Sometimes recurring crises are a by-product of the culture of your team or agency—everyone is crisis oriented, and through modeling and poor organization, crises are passed down the line. But more often, through no fault of your own, it's about you: You lack some essential skills or are emotionally overwhelmed. You're struggling with Jack because you've never been trained to assess for suicidality or you lack experience working with depressed clients. Or you have the training and knowledge, but when you look back on your sessions with Jack, you realize that he was making noises about his depression and spiraling down a few sessions ago. But your anxiety welled up, and instead of asking the hard questions, you choked and tamped down your anxiety by saying to yourself and him that that's normal, "You've just been having a hard week."

Here you need to step back, reflect, and think about the problem under the problem and the possible source of these crises. And if you decide it is at least partially about you, it's time to get the support you need—first-aid direction from your supervisor and a conversation with her about what you realize you don't know.

Not Urgent/Important

This is ideally where you want to live most of the time. You're doing your job's essential, primary tasks without the panicky deadlines or clinical crises. Certainly, primary tasks involve seeing clients, but they also include those secondary, everyday tasks that come with maintaining your job—meeting with your supervisor, attending staff meetings, completing your paperwork, filling out mileage forms, and so on. But beyond these everyday tasks, this category also includes those times when you pause to reflect and plan, focus on those larger but important tasks of setting learning goals for the next three months, or look over your caseload to think about what you are doing well and where you are struggling. Taking the time to reflect and plan is about being proactive rather than reactive.

Not Urgent/Not Important

Covey lumps into this fourth category those hallway or office catch-up conversations with colleagues, but also those end-of-day times at 4:30 on Friday when you're finished with clients, are tired from the week, and are scanning through Amazon looking at shoes. But these are also times, say I, where you occasionally but intentionally put your feet up on your desk and think big thoughts about your vision of your future or those larger goals, such as where you want to be in five years, or brainstorm what you think your clinical style and therapy are all about. Such times also offer opportunities to be creative without the driving force of just getting stuff done. Not urgent perhaps, but certainly important in the bigger picture of your career and development.

So, back to prioritizing your time based on these four categories. Here's mine: #1: not urgent/important; #2: urgent/important; #3: not urgent/not important; #4: urgent/not important.

When you look at your tasks and priorities, where do you stand and how do you wind up spending your time? Do you need to change what you are doing in some way? What do you need to get there?

CHAPTER 41

Organization One

Taking Control of Your Day

Say you have sorted through Stephen Covey's (2020) categories of tasks but found that, like it or not, a lot of your day is necessarily reactive: answering calls, texts, and emails coming at you and, obviously, responding to clients with whatever occurs at the top of the session. When too much feels out of control, you can feel burned out, that you're hustling and have no time to breathe and regroup. It is time to offset this feeling by taking control of what you can control.

Take Control over Your Client Appointments

Although many work settings allow you to set your appointments, some don't. Instead, like many medical practices, someone at the front desk looks at holes on the Outlook page and fills a slot for you, usually based on a call from a patient. This process can make for overall agency efficiency—clients don't need to do a two-step to get an appointment with you—but it may not work for you. You wind up with three depressed, potentially resistant clients, hyperactive children, or battling couples in a row in the afternoon when your energy is low. Or you're slated to see Bill, but you know from experience he's not a morning guy. Coming in after his night shift, he's sluggish, he rambles, and he can't quite grasp what you're saying, so a session in the afternoon would be more productive.

Ideally, you should schedule your own appointments: Find a time for Bill that you know is best, and break up the clump of depressed clients or hyperactive children. If you can't do your own scheduling, talk to the scheduling folks and let them know your preferences overall but even with particular clients. Unlike most doctors who deal with and think in terms of one-time sessions, you likely see folks on an ongoing basis in which your working style overall and with specific clients is important. Let your front office folks know what you need.

Dress

How you dress is part of feeling empowered. My next day's planning includes looking at my client list and deciding how to dress. If, for example, I have a couple or individual adult coming in for the first time, I'll wear a tie or a jacket—to set that all-important first impression. And if I'm feeling a bit sluggish or a bit anxious about meeting that CEO, I may dress up and wear my power suit. But if I have a day filled with teens, I might dress down—not quite as formal and hopefully not uptight and rigid. Deciding how to dress does not mean you change your clothes in the bathroom between appointments, but that you consider expectations, what the client needs to feel comfortable and safe, or what you need to feel less anxious. Map it out ahead of time, like the night before. Look at the day's caseload and decide what type of dress will make a good presentation.

Build in Time for Paperwork and for Returning Phone Calls

You hate paperwork; I hate paperwork; everyone hates paperwork. But it isn't going away. I've known a lot of therapists—experienced and less experienced—who struggle with it. Figure out your problem with paperwork, and resolve it. Feeling pressured by paperwork or not getting it done is usually driven by underlying issues—that you don't understand how to work the in-house record software or that your schedule is too tight with client sessions, and you have no time to fit it in. Or it is more about your attitude—it's boring, your ADHD kicks in, or you're perfectionistic, and a simple progress note can take you a half hour to craft.

If completing paperwork is about the system, speak up and help your IT person know what doesn't work or get training to manage paperwork better. If the issue is about not having time, talk to your supervisor. If the issue is about you, tackle you.

In the meantime, it helps to dedicate time to doing your paperwork. I've worked at agencies where folks literally had the last hour or half hour of the day to do paperwork, or Friday afternoons were set aside for doing paperwork and no clients were scheduled. Some workplaces have clinicians write their notes during or near the end of each session. Find out what the workplace can provide and decide what might work best. The danger is that if you don't tackle this problem head-on, it will be a constant source of stress and anxiety.

Check Your Mood and Plan Accordingly

Because you're not working by yourself repairing computers or car engines, your mood on a given day impacts clients. If you wake up in a lousy mood because you didn't sleep well, because the baby was waking up, because you had a late-night argument with your partner that is still lingering, because you woke up obsessing at 3:00 A.M., take note. Know that you might be overreactive to the couple battling the similar arguments you had with your partner. Know that your energy is low because of lack of sleep, and you may need to grab that cup of coffee or walk around the building before you see energetic Jake at 4:00. Your mood may change over the day—you make up with your partner during your lunch break or the coffee kicks in and you feel okay at 4:00—but check in with yourself and gauge your mood throughout the day.

Have Plans in Advance

You have a new couple arriving on Tuesday or a new client on Thursday with an eating disorder, and you're not yet comfortable with couple therapy or with eating disorders. If some clients and issues create a background anxiety for you, step back and map your plans. Map out on Monday what you want to cover with the couple; schedule a quick check-in with your supervisor first thing on Thursday morning to create a preliminary plan for your Thursday client.

The theme here is countering the reactive nature of your work by being as proactive as possible. Figure out what you need, what works, and experiment. Find the right organizational and personal mix that works best for you.

CHAPTER 42

Organization Two

Setting Priorities

In the previous chapter, we talked about specific ways to make your day feel less reactive and anxious and more productive. Here we look at ways of organizing your week to manage other tasks besides client appointments and to set some priorities.

Here's an eight-step approach that I've suggested to clients over the years and have used myself. It works well for me, and may well help you be more in control.

1. Map Out the Five Most Important Things You Need to Get Done in the Next Week

Ideally, you do this task on Sunday night. Why? Because once you get to your office on Monday morning, you're likely to go on reactive mode or autopilot. You get caught up in the flurry of the actual workweek and feel overwhelmed by the demands coming at you. Doing this task on Sunday gives you the time and space to rationally look ahead and sort out your priorities. By limiting the to-do list to five tasks rather than to 50, you push against your anxiety that tells you everything is important and helps you not feel overwhelmed.

2. Map Out the Three Things You Need to Do Each Next Day

Your Sunday night to-do list gives you the big picture, but you need to next break it down into smaller, doable tasks. Here you sit down with yourself on Monday night to map out the three tasks you absolutely need to do on Tuesday that are part of the big five. For instance, you may decide to outline your self-evaluation due on Friday, finish the progress notes of the clients you saw on Thursday and Friday, or contact the caseworker at social services. If it helps, put a sticky note on your computer or a note on Outlook or your phone—something you can write down and then check off.

Why Monday night and not Tuesday morning? Again, you are engaging your rational brain rather than your anxious/reactive brain to proactively map out what you realistically can accomplish in a certain amount of time. And by deciding on the tasks the evening before, you are also priming your brain to hit the ground running on Tuesday morning, rather than waking up, deciding you're tired because you didn't sleep well, and saying to yourself that whatever you thought you should do today, you'll do tomorrow.

3. Do Hard Stuff First for 30 Minutes

We all tend to procrastinate about tasks that seem hard—generally because they are overwhelming or boring. Try tackling what seems most difficult first—both to get those tasks out of the way and to increase your tolerance for the hard stuff. Do the progress notes, leave a message or send an email to the social services contact, or map out your thoughts about your evaluation. Do the hard stuff first, so you're not tempted to put it off because you are rushed or tired later in the day. And you want to do it for 30 minutes, so you don't sabotage yourself with unrealistic expectations of having to work yourself to death until it's done.

4. Take a Fifteen-Minute Break

Taking a break is important if you are doing a longer task. The key here is to time the break so you don't wander off—check your email before your first appointment but never come back; chat with a colleague about a case and leave no time to circle back. Taking a break is a way of getting mentally and emotionally recentered, not a reason to push off what you need to do.

5. Do Another 30-Minute Round

You've had your break; give the task one more 30-minute round if you need more time to finish it. One caveat: If being a perfectionist is what is driving you, take the risk of stopping and saying to yourself that what you've done is good enough.

6. Give Yourself a Reward

Treat yourself to another cup of coffee or tea, chat with your colleague, enjoy your lunch, or look up restaurants for dinner on Friday night. Solidify accomplishing the hard stuff with positive reinforcements.

7. Move On to the Easier Tasks

With the most challenging stuff out of the way, you now can tackle other items that are less overwhelming or require less focus. You can continue to do blocks of time with timed breaks, but your day isn't done until you cross these items off your list. Give yourself another reward at the end of the day for accomplishing your . . . day. Plot out the next day before you go to bed.

8. Be Careful of All-or-Nothing Thinking

Resist the temptation of looking at your watch at 2:00 and saying, "Wow, it's already late, the day is shot; I'll finish the rest of the stuff tomorrow." Stay on track by staying on track and not finding excuses to put your tasks off.

Give this approach a try. Again, it's about being proactive, learning to do the hard before the easy, not being emotionally driven, and rewiring your brain.

PART IV

YOUR CAREER

Let's move out of the workplace, step back, and look at your work from a larger viewpoint—your career. We can think of our career as moving through four stages—from novice to independent practitioner—and this progression is what we walk through in this part. By knowing the characteristics of and opportunities at each stage, you'll hopefully not only feel reassured but can also anticipate the changes that might be coming. But first, let's see how you think about your work.

CHAPTER 43

Your Work

A Job, a Career, a Calling

Leben and *arbeiten,* love and work, said Freud about what drives life. Love can be fickle, somewhat out of our control. But work, that's something we can control—sort of. You have already chosen your career path and worked hard to gain the skills you need to move forward in your life. But before you just march ahead, pause and ask yourself about the role of work in your life. Basically, you have three possible perspectives.

1. My Work Is a Job

You enjoy what you do, and are good at it, but regardless of your title or your tasks, your job is your job. You're not one to work overtime or wake up in the middle of the night worrying about the next day. Other things are more important in your life—your kids, your family, your passion for rebuilding old cars, or playing the saxophone in a local band. This job is the best way to make money and maintain your lifestyle; it's not on the top of your list; it's a means, not an end.

2. My Work Is My Career

Yes, your job is a job, but it is something more. It is more than what you do, but who you are. You may have a vision—of eventually being the best therapist in a 100-mile radius or being known as an amazing teacher. Or your ultimate goal is less clear, the path forward shrouded in mist, but there are the beginnings of a path nonetheless. This is the first step in becoming dedicated to your work.

3. My Work Is a Calling

Your work becomes a significant part of who you are. This is what you were born to do; your values and beliefs make you an advocate for the poor, the abused, or the mentally ill. It's not about money or about moving ahead, but about having a purpose—you do what you do because you need to do it. You really don't have any other choice.

Many of us rotate through some combination of all of these perspectives, depending on the day, our stress level, and where we are in our lives. For others, their perspectives on the job, the career, or the calling may take hold for years or decades, but then slowly or suddenly shift: career replaces job, kids replace career, calling replaces career. Our priorities change because we and what we need from our lives change.

Successfully navigating these changes is about realizing that they may occur and periodically stepping back and reflecting on the role of your work in your life. If you don't, if you continue to run on autopilot, it becomes all too easy to lose the relationship between your work and your life. Instead, you fall into the everyday grind and continue to do what you do because it's what you do; you've lost your vision or have given up and feel it is too late to change. You reconcile yourself to a life you are given rather than to a life you can create.

But you don't want to give up on creating your life. So, step back and ask: What role does work play in your life right now? Is it fulfilling what you need most? What do you need or want to change?

CHAPTER 44

One Year Out

Moving from Content to Process

In earlier chapters, we talked about transitions and clinical challenges—about the familiar sources of anxiety that often occur at the beginning of your career, that stage where you realize what you don't know. Some clinicians don't move past this stage in their jobs. They find that the work doesn't fit their interests and personality, or that they prefer to work with different populations or in another environment—in schools as guidance counselors or in hospitals where they are part of a team—and they leave.

But for others, the problem isn't about the work not fitting them, but more about feeling that they can't fit the work. Despite their best efforts, they stay overwhelmed, never settle, and begin to believe that they'll never be good enough. Rather than realizing that the problem isn't their lack of ability but their anxiety, rather than pushing back against it and clarifying expectations or requesting the training they need, they believe what their anxiety is telling them: that the only way to avoid feeling anxious is to simply do more and be more perfect. So, they bail and look for a setting where the expectations and stress seem more manageable. They haven't realized that those first few months or first year are the worst it will get, and they haven't given themselves a good enough chance or gotten the support they need, and so they leave the clinical field prematurely.

From Content to Process

"During the past year, I have gained new knowledge about the middle phases of treatment. I've learned more about my difficulty confronting clients, but I am learning to use clients' reactions to me to effect change. Rather than being a friend, I now often present myself as a teammate to the families I work with. But the negative side of my joining skills is my tendency to feel responsible for the family. I need to develop enough distance to help individuals learn how to take care of themselves as well as prevent my own burnout. I still struggle with developing confidence in my professional self."

Paula is writing this reflection as part of her self-evaluation at the end of her first year on the job. Like most new graduates, she had a challenging start where she felt overwhelmed, filled with impostor syndrome, and constantly worried about her performance. But in the past few months Paula has turned a corner—she has begun to settle and is moving away from the accommodating, overly responsible stance of those first months when she tried to befriend her clients, and that, in turn, led her to feel burned out.

Paula is aware that she has changed, and we can see this awareness in what she writes and in the language she uses. She defines herself as a teammate with clients—you and me against the problem—connoting a more even playing field; she is no longer one-down, scrambling to please. Paula acknowledges her continuing tendency to be overresponsible, but she now has a choice because she is aware of it. Now she has the opportunity to recognize this tendency, pull back, and change her reaction as it is unfolding.

And it is the unfolding that Paula can now focus on. This is the important part of her self-evaluation: She can use the clients' reactions to shape her own in the session. Rather than focusing on and being overwhelmed by content—the what—she is becoming aware of the how—the process. This is huge; a paradigm shift. Rather than feeling the pressure to somehow fix all of the clients' content—those problems *out there* in their lives—which Paula has little or no control over, she realizes that her only impact is what she says and does within the confines of the clinical session. Just as she can alter her response to her clients in the session, she can now help them change their response to the problems that erupt in their lives.

Don't Know What You Know

This shift from content to process is characteristic of the second stage of clinical development. But also another part of this stage is a shift from "I know what I don't know" to "I don't know what I know." Here you know stuff, you've gotten your sea legs, but you are inconsistent. You have a good session one week but a difficult one the following week, and you're unsure why. Or you do a good job with some clients but struggle with others. You've learned a lot, but your knowledge and skills are integrated, not unlike on the behavioral level of toddlers who may stumble and fall or trip over themselves, but over time fall less as they become stronger and learn to work their muscles.

And because you are settled, have leaned into your supervisor and colleagues, and are less anxious, this is a great time to focus on fine-tuning your awareness of the microprocess: to pay attention to the unfolding process, to learn to hear the dismissiveness when you interpret, to step back and read the climate in the room, to notice those transference cues so you can craft what you say so as not to trigger negative reactions and stay in lockstep with the client. This can be an exciting and productive time when you realize that you can shape what happens in a session because you are more aware of what is happening around you.

Seduced by Intimacy

Like the first stage, where there is the danger that you might not be able to contain your anxiety, this stage has its own danger, namely, dependency. At this point you may have clients who have been in treatment for a long while; they have become reliant on you as their primary source of support. But what you both share is the intimacy of the relationship itself, and that intimacy is seductive. Any active problem solving has been superseded by the client feeling comforted by seeing you week after week. And the same happens on your side—you see Ms. Jones at 2:00 on Tuesday because you see Ms. Jones at 2:00 on Tuesday. There's a bit of going on autopilot, but also you look forward to seeing her. She appreciates what you do, and you appreciate the intimacy and the appreciation. The danger is the autopilot, the losing sight of goals, the dependency defined as "good relationship, no change." Rather than taking a more assertive role or terminating therapy, you don't.

If you suspect a dependency may be happening, you need to talk with your supervisor. You want to periodically step back and ask yourself and your client whether or not you are still on track and whether and how therapy needs to be continued. Be honest with yourself and your client about the process and goals of the therapy.

If you are at or are approaching this stage in your career, what do you need most to increase your awareness of what is unfolding within sessions? Now that you have some traction and can survey the larger landscape of your work, what impasses arise, and what problems or types of clients do you most struggle with? If you are still feeling flooded with content or taking on too much responsibility for the outcome, are you aware of when these reactions occur? If not, how can you be more attuned? What support or training do you need to realize these limits on your own impact?

CHAPTER 45

Moving On

Coming into Your Power

In the original *Star Wars* movies, our hero, Luke Skywalker, is training under Yoda to be a Jedi Knight. In the middle of his training, he learns that his friends, Princess Leia and Han Solo, have been captured and decides that he needs to leave to go save them. But both Yoda and Obi-Wan caution him that he is at a fragile time in his training—that the forces of the dark would will tempt him, that although he has learned so much, he can't yet control the power he has gained.

Let's return to Paula, the clinician we met in the last chapter. She too is at a fragile and pivotal point in her training. Again, let's look at her self-evaluation, but after two years have passed. Here's what she has to say:

"I'd like to find better ways to handle my anger toward clients. . . . Because of the anxiety that change arouses, change is not always accepted or attempted by clients. I must remember to help clients take responsibility for their choices about change and realize that all clients are not ready to make the changes necessary. . . . I feel I have a greater sense of my power and a greater awareness of my own anger. I worry less about their reactions."

Do you hear the change? If you find similarities between this clinician's feelings and your current feeling toward your own competence, you are in a new stage: "Don't know what you don't know." What does this mean? You know a good deal, but there are things you don't know, and you are often unaware of these blind spots. The corollary is that you think you know everything. And with this realization comes a shift in role. You change from being accommodating, doing too much, and being overresponsible to acknowledging and, at times, resenting that you've been doing too much of the heavy lifting and are frustrated that clients aren't working as hard as you are. At this point, our clinician refers to therapy as a choice, and she concludes that some clients are not ready to make the necessary changes.

What comes with this stage is a more proactive stance. With increased skill and confidence, therapists have a clearer sense of what needs to be done, rather than building around what clients offer. But this stage is also the time when some clinicians can become impatient and notice resistance. While Paula is able to say that some clients may not be ready for therapy, other clinicians might frame a client's reaction more stringently—if clients are unwilling to work, their treatment is done, and they can be suddenly terminated. And in these more extreme cases, clinicians can be inflexible and can seem haughty and arrogant. If clients are not attuned to their approach or follow their suggestions, they are seen as resistant and cast aside.

This unawareness of blind spots is not just limited to the mental health profession. You are not alone; these blind spots and arrogance infect other fields as well. In looking at political scandals, for example, notice that it is not the freshman congressperson who gets caught for laundering campaign money, but the senior congresswoman who thinks she's immune—again the blind spots—but this is a dangerous time on an ethical level. Clinicians can succumb to sexual abuse of clients and find some way of rationalizing their behavior, or they develop areas of conflict and dual relationships. For example, you ask your client, who works as a carpenter, to give you an estimate for building a deck and rationalize, "What's the big deal?" Or supervisors start to have attitude problems from individual staff people who are slacking on paperwork, complaining about policies, or shuffling agency clients into their budding private practices. Fortunately, most clinicians don't go there, but if it's going to happen, it's likely to occur at this stage.

But what also flares up at this stage is restlessness—growing out of your job or your supervisor. You want to learn something more, or you are burned out on the type of work you've been doing. Some practitioners take trainings in a totally new approach—change from psychodynamic to cognitive-behavioral therapy (CBT) or to bodywork practice.

Or they switch from clinical work to administration. Or they leave the field altogether and set up a business building guitars or selling real estate. They're done with living in a world of problems, being on call, or worrying about what Sam may or may not do when mowing their grass or making the bed on the weekend.

This is a time of empowerment, but as with all adult stages of life, the beginnings are shaky; some new feelings and needs are not yet controlled.

CHAPTER 46

A Voice of Your Own

At some point, you move through and past those earlier stages and challenges—the "know what you don't know," "don't know what you know," and "don't know what you don't know." You reach the stage where you "know what you know." Let's return to Paula, our clinician, once more to see what's changed. She starts by describing her view of therapy and client motivation:

"I believe that clients need to be motivated to change but realize that what seems like initial resistance is often just anxiety regarding the unfamiliar process of therapy itself. . . . When anxious or stressed, I notice how I sometimes still fall back into my saving mode or react passive-aggressively. But I'm much more sensitive to the signs that I am getting stressed, and realize they're telling me I need to take care of myself. . . . Supervision has gone beyond ensuring the quality of my work to helping me expand my sense of self and professional growth. I would like to take a greater leadership role in the community regarding mental health and children. I feel that I have much that I can teach and give."

Notice the change from the previous stage: Paula is no longer talking about anger. Earlier, she felt that some clients were not ready for therapy, and that was their choice; she now realizes she needs to cut them some slack. She acknowledges that she can slip into being overresponsible (old coping methods die hard), but can not only put the brakes on it, but also recognize her overresponsibility as a sign that she is getting burned out. Paula is expanding her view of herself and can use her clinical strengths and self-confidence to envision a future of greater opportunities.

To know what you know is to accept that you don't know everything, and accept that that's okay. Gone is the arrogance of the previous stage. You've settled on a style and clinical approach that works for you. You've realized what you're good at and enjoy doing without feeling the pressure to do more or be all things to all people. How long does it take to get to this point? Our clinician was ten years out of graduate school when she wrote these thoughts. Getting to this stage may take several more years for some clinicians, and probably less time for only a few.

Reaching this stage doesn't mean personal growth is over, although there is always a danger that you would conclude that it is. Like some tenured professors who teach the same courses year after year, no longer do any research and essentially coast, some clinicians act the same way. They settle into their clinical routines; they log what training hours they need to keep up their licenses, but they don't explore new approaches or techniques. While their clinical style is still effective for many clients, it becomes less flexible. They may downgrade their work to that of a "job" rather than a career or calling; they save their energy for interests outside of work.

But with any luck, that won't be you. Rather, you'll continue to explore and grow. I moved into administration, then into private practice and training. You might go into program development; challenge yourself by working in a different setting and with different populations (clients in hospitals, prisons, and schools); get out of straight clinical work and become a life coach; serve your community by going on local radio shows; speak to Optimist Clubs about children; volunteer at the community free clinic; or become famous by working up your specialties and teaching, training others, or consulting, writing articles and books, or creating your own YouTube videos.

And as you age, your priorities will likely change. That midlife crisis may stimulate you to go for the high-end administrative job or write that book, or it may do the opposite, cause you to want to spend more time with your kids before they scatter. Or you might decide that you love the interaction with clients and just make some technical changes that deepen your skills, insights, and wisdom. You're also fortunate to work at a job that you can continue to do as long as you want—you're not a construction worker who worries that his knees or back are wearing out and sidelining him.

So, where do you envision yourself, your work, and your life in the next ten or 20 years?

CHAPTER 47

How to Use Trainings

Some trainings that agencies require may or may not seem relevant to your everyday work—in basic first aid, in handling hazardous materials, in diversity awareness, or in record-keeping software. There are other trainings that your licensing board may require that are important to maintaining your professional self—a set number of hours in ethics each year or getting continuing education credits (CEUs) in supervision. And then there are those trainings that deal directly with your clinical work.

The kind and quality of clinical training you get may be driven less by your particular needs than by other factors, such as agency requirements, the financial cost, and time out of the office. Rather than sending you to that three-day play therapy training in Chicago that, with transportation and hotels, will run over $1,000, your supervisor is happy to send you to a day-long workshop offered by the state mental health office that only costs $20 a head, and you can carpool with your colleagues. Your supervisor sees it as a perk; you see it as interesting and as a chance to get out of the office for a day.

Or perhaps your agency brings in someone from the outside to train on some approach that the agency is planning on offering as a new program or as a means of reaching a new population—trainings in internal family systems, in new models for working with addictions, or in conducting parenting groups for clients referred by social services. Again, helpful stuff that certainly enhances your skill set, but may or may not fit your current needs and interests.

Although financial considerations, practical options, and agency priorities are always part of the mix, decisions about trainings should ideally be reached based on your current needs as a professional. Here's where you sit down with yourself and then your supervisor and survey the state of your clinical work. You link trainings into your six-month or yearly goals. What populations, problems, or skills are you struggling with—young children and play therapy, violent couples, teens who are self-harming? And what are your passions—working with trauma victims or with current approaches to pain management? You're proactive and deliberate about what you need rather than taking what you get (or choosing the workshop near your brother because you can crash on the couch and save yourself or the agency money).

Regardless of what the training will focus on, you need to decide what *type* of training fills that educational hole. Because trainings come in all shapes and sizes, here's a quick guide to help you find the format that suits your needs best.

Several-Hour or All-Day Trainings

Sometimes these formats are built into a multiday conference. By attending one of these conferences, you not only have a wide variety of workshops to choose from, but you also get to meet clinicians from outside your area, get to talk shop, and even get to party in the evening (unless you have to leave to go to your brother's). Some of these two-day workshops are stand-alone, either live and on-site or online.

These shorter workshops are great for introducing you to an area of therapy you've been curious about—EMDR, internal family systems, or attachment disorders and their impact on intimate relationships—and where you'll get a mix of theory and techniques. They also can provide helpful updates on topics in which you already have a foundation, like the latest information on legal and liability issues or current research on the effects of trauma on the brain.

The downside is that these workshops are short. You walk out with plenty of excitement but with only enough information and skill to be dangerous. You've stuck your toes in the water, but if you want to reach any level of competence in working with the new ideas, you need to learn more. You may decide to sign up for one or several weekend-long workshops, read the presenter's book, or better yet, convince your supervisor to allow you and a couple of colleagues who also attended the workshop to form a study group, where you all read the book or watch videos and take baby steps to apply what you're learning and learn from each other's experiences.

Two- or Three-Day Certification Programs

These programs are one step up from the several-hour or day-long workshop format. Many training companies are using this model, usually an all-day Friday-to-Sunday format, and the topics are numerous—CBT, EMDR, working with sexual addictions and various forms of anxiety, clinical supervision. You walk out with a paper saying you've completed a course and are certified. What you get while there is not only the theory, but also lots of demonstrations and exercises to try out the new skills. Obviously, there's more to learn, and certainly, much more practice is needed, but in the end, you're not quite as dangerous; you can usually begin applying what you learn right away.

Long-Term Trainings

You can take another step up the training ladder by enrolling in intensive training programs. They may involve attending a day-long seminar monthly for three years; signing up for a year-long program that meets weekly for three hours; or participating in a mix of long weekends, outside readings, a certain number of clinical hours, or having clients using the approach along with supervised support.

These programs are about delving deeper. Like an apprenticeship, they help to develop your skills, and you can add a new lens to your work. You get support from others in the program whom you can get to know and befriend. You may run with the approach and use it more or less exclusively, or it becomes something you integrate into your unique clinical style over time. The downside is higher costs, taking time off work, or spending extra time on weekends working rather than going to your kid's soccer game.

Cotherapy, Observation, and Supervision

Not all training has to feel like training, and it doesn't have to involve metal chairs and squishing against the guy next to you. Sometimes it's good to think outside the box and keep it simple—a training for one: you. You feel you are weak in couple or family therapy or lack skills in play therapy or working with teens. Here you ask Jane if you can be a cotherapist with one or two of her couples or families. You tag along with Mark when he goes out to an elementary school and works with a child in play therapy. You sit in a corner and observe, or if there happens to be a one-way mirror in your office space, you take advantage of it. Or you want to learn more about object-relationships approaches, so you talk to your supervisor, who may direct you to Teresa down the hall or to someone outside the practice that she knows is experienced in this treatment style. You do your readings, use them as a temporary mentor, then watch what other experienced clinicians do and handle cases on your own that they help you deconstruct.

Depending on your needs and goals, this kind of professional development can be short or long term. The advantage here is that you learn in maybe the best possible way—seeing someone else in action who can model what to do and then can explain how to do it, and eventually help you do what she does. This kind of training can be a powerful learning tool and experience. It's a form of apprenticeship that's worked forever.

About trainings and your clinical development, bear this in mind: When you're starting out, going to a bunch of two-hour workshops at a large conference may be stimulating, but it can also leave you feeling confused or even self-critical and knowing what you don't know. Cotherapy and supervision may provide a good middle ground as you feel more stable and secure in your knowledge. Intensive training may come later when you have a firm foundation, know what you know, and understand what you want to learn. Trying these programs at this stage not only allows you to build upon a solid base so that you don't feel rattled, but because of your experience allows you to integrate these new ideas—sure, they're talking about *x*, but that's just a variation of what I do when I do *y*; I can combine *x* with *y*, and for these clients that combination would be a new and powerful form of treatment.

Try to see training as something more than clocking in CEU hours or getting out of the office. It's a way of staying energized and skilled to better serve your clients, feeling less anxious and more competent, reaching your own clinical goals, and becoming that clinician you envision yourself becoming.

What is it you need to learn now? What are you curious about and want to possibly explore in the future? What format works the best for you?

CHAPTER 48

When You Outgrow Your Job

There will come a day when you notice that something has changed about your relationship with your work. The anxiety you remember feeling about new clients and new problems and struggling to keep up with paperwork is still there sometimes, but it's low level. You have those days feeling a sense of dread, but it's different from the dread of burnout. Earlier in your career it was combined with exhaustion or the tiredness of constantly feeling on edge and reacting and dealing; your escape fantasies were about quitting and going into IT repair or a simpler life working at the post office. This is a different dread, more along the lines of "same sh*t, different day"—one driven by boredom, perhaps a feeling of being stuck or trapped, and certainly a restlessness.

You're outgrowing your job, which is no surprise. If you have been doing your job and your supervisor has been doing her job—supporting, teaching, and challenging you—you naturally gained skills and confidence from accumulating experience. Your restlessness is a sign that you're not the same clinician or person that you were a few years ago, that the job no longer fits you. What to do?

You have several options, and all are predicated on your personality, overall goals, and opportunities.

Change Your Process

It's estimated that 40% of our days run on habit (Duhigg, 2014) and, no doubt, if you're honest, you're aware that habits have even bled into your clinical work. If you're stuck in a rut, the first step to getting out of it might be looking at how you conduct your sessions and trying out a minor change. Rather than saying, "How was your week?" as soon as your client sits down, maybe say, "Okay, I want to know more about what you said at the end of the last session about breaking up with Bill." Or, rather than wading through the same format of catch-ups, shake it up. Ask about something new—recent dreams, unknown family members—or do something new—a guided imagery exercise. Or just sit there and see what happens.

This option isn't about clinical goals but about clinical process, energy, and spontaneity. Therapy, after all, is about change. Bring it into the therapy session.

Change Your Caseload

Your caseload is half kids or depressed clients. You know what to do, have clear treatment maps, but the sameness is wearing you down. A simple fix here may be to change your day—fill the other 50% with folks who force you to not go on autopilot and to use a different part of your brain—and talk with your supervisor.

If you talk about wanting to change your caseload or feeling burned out, a good supervisor will hear the warning signs of restlessness and might take your requests seriously; she may realize that there is a danger that you might bolt. Bolting is often part of agency-based work, but it's hell for a supervisor who constantly needs to recruit and build up her staff. You have some clout. See what she says, what she can do.

Look for Intensive Training

You're not bored with your clients; you're bored with yourself. You're doing the same thing all the time, thinking the same way, and changing your process isn't enough. You need to challenge your thinking.

This is a good opportunity to go for some training. Here you want to listen to your gut. If you have any wisp of curiosity about something, however outside your comfort zone it may seem, explore. Are you tired of working with adults and have that wisp of interest in play therapy? Always wondering what object-relations therapy is all about? Intrigued by the notion of hypnosis? Check it out. This curiosity is not about play therapy or hypnosis but about nurturing that tiny flame of change, paying attention to your inner gut and voices.

The next step might be to do something small to investigate a new interest—explore an online course or webinar, a weekend training, or the options we discussed in the last chapter. Get your feet wet. And as discussed in the previous chapter, with your accumulated experience, you are at the best time in your clinical development to understand and use what you hear. And if there is something that ignites you, consider a more extended training. Talk to your supervisor; make the case that additional training will improve your practice (and keep you at the agency). Ask if your agency can subsidize the training either with financial assistance or give you time off.

Change Supervisors

This is third on the list because, in many settings, and as we discussed before, changing supervisors is often not an option. In small, often rural agencies, the career ladder is your job, your supervisor's job; we're done. But sometimes, this is an option. The reason to change supervisors? Hopefully, it's not because you simply can't get along; you've tackled that problem in the first year of employment. But if, several years later, you realize that you've reached the limits of your knowledge and skills with your supervisor or you want to explore a different clinical approach that your supervisor is not experienced in, these are good reasons to try and shift gears.

So you bring up your need for change with your supervisor. Be clear about your goals: Are you wanting someone who overall has a different approach—say, Adam, who runs the adult team but is well versed in object-relations approaches—versus having Megan, who knows play therapy inside and out and can supervise you on a few cases? Pulling back from supervisors can often seem a bigger deal than it needs to be (remember Freud and Jung—Jung tried to pull away by talking about archetypes, and Freud was threatened and then literally cut off their relationship). To avoid having your supervisor feel threatened in any way, help her understand your desire for change as a need for growth rather than as a betrayal and abandonment; work out the details related to her concerns about quality control. You may be able to switch to Adam or Megan, and the switch may resolve your clinical itch.

Look for a New Job

A new job may be in your current workplace—applying for a supervisory position, a new grant program director—or outside it. Go for it.

Looking for a new job is about moving forward, so you're not feeling trapped and are able to gain perspective. Pursuing a promotion allows you to see what the next level in your organization is like; applying for jobs with different agencies gives you a sense of varying tasks and skills and diverse work cultures—more laid-back, more or less team focused, more or less supportive, more variety or less.

By exploring this way, you have something to bounce off of, which in turn can help you better define what you need and want most—a clinical challenge, a simple do-something-different, or a better work climate. You may find a job that better suits your current needs or not. But if you don't, you've gained a new perspective; by checking out other opportunities, you can look at your current position in a new light. You're likely to mentally and emotionally return not with a sense of resignation but with more energy and appreciation.

Whatever you decide to do, the underlying driver is your evolution—that, like it or not, you're going to change in some way, even if you do nothing different at all. The challenge is creating a new box in your life when the old ones don't fit rather than squeezing yourself into the old box that no longer works. Your ongoing challenge is revamping your life to fit who you are now.

CHAPTER 49

Transitions

Clinician to Supervisor

On the first day of my graduate school supervision course, the professor confidently said that it was likely that all of us would be supervisors in two years. "Yeah, right," I smirked, but he was right. Two years into my job, there I was supervising a newly graduated, newly hired clinician. What I wound up doing is what many new supervisors do: I'd ask my colleague what she wanted to talk about; she would present a case; we talked about what she planned to do, or that she didn't know what to do; and then I, in my infinite wisdom, gave her suggestions that she'd dutifully write down. She left (I like to think) feeling a bit of relief; I left wondering what the hell I was doing.

I've since realized that being a supervisor is more than being that senior clinician I was pretending to be. Like therapy, the world of clinical supervision is multifaceted, composed of various models and skill sets. The one I learned in graduate school is what I call the "multiple-hats" model. The core concept here is that as a supervisor, your job requires you to wear the different hats—teacher, supporter, quality controller, administrator, community representative—that make up your job. According to this model, a good supervisor is one who knows what hat to wear at any given time, can switch hats fluidly, and be comfortable in wearing each one. This model was likely the one used at my school because it works well in public agencies.

But two other models of clinical supervision are also in use: one based on specific clinical approaches and the other based on developmental stages. The clinically based models are diverse. If you are psychodynamically oriented, supervision focuses on helping the clinician learn to think and practice in terms of psychodynamic concepts—looking at patient history and unresolved childhood issues and sorting out transference and countertransference issues. In contrast, cognitive-behavioral supervision focuses on how the clients' thoughts and behaviors, and your own, can shape the clients' treatment and the process of the therapy itself. Similarly, other supervision models are based on object-relations, attachment, and solution-focused therapy; the list goes on and on.

Development models, on the other hand, consider how clinicians grow and change as they gain knowledge and experience; in this book, this model has been the basis of our discussion about the various stages in your career. You need to anticipate, adapt, and accommodate to where the supervisee is at and where the person is going. Just as in the "multiple-hats" approach, you want to switch hats easily; you don't want to be doing the same thing with Ebony, a new clinician, on day 300 that you did on day one, nor do you want to do the same supervision as you would do with Victor, who has eight years' experience. And like the multiple-hats approach, this model works particularly well if you supervise several therapists with different levels of experience.

Whatever model you train in or settle upon, you have two primary jobs as a supervisor: providing quality control—making sure that the agency's clients and the community are receiving quality services given the experience level of your staff and that disastrous mistakes are avoided—and supporting your supervisees so that they only provide good or good-enough services but that they feel supported and that they grow as clinicians.

Three Mistakes to Avoid

There are several mistakes that are easy to make and avoid. One is spoon-feeding. Spoon-feeding is essentially doing remote-control clinical work. Allen, for example, is a new clinician who comes to supervision and says he is struggling with Josh, a depressed older gentleman, or with Mateo, a child with ADHD. He can make a diagnosis, but he is unsure about what the treatment plan should be. So you step up and give him a detailed step-by-step plan about what to do with Josh or Mateo in his next session. Allen walks out happy. Not only does he not have to worry about what to do, but he doesn't have to worry about making some big mistake. Even if the session doesn't go well, it's not because he screwed up—he was, after all, only doing what you suggested. And you too as his supervisor are also less anxious: By giving him clear directives, you can rest easy—not wake up at 3:00 A.M. worrying if Allen will do something disastrous.

This pattern is powerful and seductive because you and Allen are colluding: By spoon-feeding, you reduce each other's anxiety by increasing control. The danger here is that after a few supervisory sessions like this one, spoon-feeding can quickly become a set format, what supervision is about.

The cost to Allen is that he trades his lower anxiety for clinical growth. Rather than helping him figure out how and why he gets stuck and find a solution that fits his skills and personality, he doesn't. Instead, he begins leaning more and more in your direction and never turns the corner on learning to think for himself. And there is a larger danger: Because of the parallel process, how you treat Allen dribbles down to how Allen treats his clients. He tells his clients what to do about their problems, which encourages clients to become dependent on him. They, like him, never learn to solve them on their own.

Don't do this.

Another common and related mistake is that you don't micromanage Allen but spend most of your supervisory sessions discussing his clients: you talk about Josh and his childhood; you brainstorm about the source of Mateo's ADHD. While your insights may initially help Allen learn how to think about Josh and Mateo and their problems, if you continue to instruct Allen, you are again essentially doing remote control clinical work. You are being that senior clinician passing on your wisdom and containing your anxiety by focusing on the clients rather than on the clinician's thinking about his clients. Again, this pattern is easy to fall into but is again one that prevents Allen from thinking on his own and developing his style.

Finally, mistake number three is that you disregard the developmental process. You do with Allen what you essentially do with all your supervisees, regardless of their experience and clients. You're doing cookie-cutter supervision. It helps you reduce your anxiety (it's familiar, after all), but you're not tailoring it to the needs of the clients or clinicians. The danger here is that your supervisees will either replicate this approach with their clients—creating a workplace climate that is rigid and limiting—one that your clinicians will eventually outgrow. They've learned what you have to offer, feel a need for something more, and realize it isn't going to come from you.

All of these mistakes are understandable traps to fall into but are ineffective ways of coping with the transition from clinician to supervisor. Supervision requires a different mindset that goes beyond a rigid clinical focus. What you need instead is training in clinical supervision itself. If you aren't getting it or can't get it from your workplace, take the initiative to find it yourself.

Moving Up the Chain

But if these challenges are not enough, there are more. Your supervisor has hired a clinician with similar clinical experience as you have, or worse, one who is older. You're feeling intimidated. Or you've been promoted from the ranks and now need to supervise your previous friends and colleagues. Here you need to lean on your current supervisor to help navigate this new set of anxieties, to help you move from being part of the pack to lead dog with new responsibilities and goals.

But there's also a change in your everyday duties. You need to have ways of ensuring quality control—checking records, staying on top of the status of at-risk clients, checking progress notes in preparation for the audit coming down the pike. You have to worry about and develop budgets; your supervisor is now asking you what candidate to hire or whether applying for a grant is a good idea. Or you're serving on an interagency committee on which you not only feel like the new kid on the block and are a bit intimidated by the older, more experienced people in the room but by having to make suggestions about the community and agency that are way outside your clinical comfort zone.

This is a bit about faking-it-till-you-make-it, and just like when you first started out, the antidote is getting the support and training you need. You're a newbie once again, albeit in a different role. As with all transitions, your inclination is to do more of what you've already been doing, and the challenge is to move beyond old ways of working. Be aware of your anxiety and ask for what you need from your supervisor—training on preparing budgets, overall support, clear directives about supervising your former colleagues, and concrete feedback on how to avoid spoon-feeding. And if you can't get what you need from your supervisor, again look elsewhere—supervisors outside your system, training from workshops and books, and perhaps even individual therapy.

Moving into a supervisory role is a difficult transition for many good reasons. Be patient with yourself. Manage your anxiety by acknowledging your anxiety and its source. Realize that making this move is about learning new skills, not revamping your clinical style or personality. Be proactive to avoid sliding into being reactive or going on autopilot.

CHAPTER 50

Going Private

We've talked about the transitions from the academic world to that first job and from beginning clinician to supervisor; now we look at our last step, the transition from public to private practice. Although you may never go in this direction but continue your career in various positions in a public or private agency system, some therapists have starting a private practice as a goal before graduating: work a few years, get the supervision, the license, and then break out. For others, the decision to go solo comes further down the line. At some point, they feel that they have outgrown their agency job and need a new challenge or are tired of the bureaucracy. Or they want to work with a different population, make more money, or to specialize. There's that well-known career question: Would you rather have power, money, or fame? From the outside, it seems that private practice can offer all three.

Regardless of the reason, the transition to private practice entails a change of environment, having different expectations, and embracing a new role that can be a challenge as you shift gears and get your sea legs. Here are some of those common hurdles and tips for moving forward.

The Emotional Terrain

When I decided to go into private practice, I had been at my agency for eighteen years. I was known in the community and had a good reputation, but still, I worried that I wouldn't have any clients and that what

I thought was a good reputation would be a paper dragon. I felt something I hadn't felt since I started, namely, performance pressure. I never had to worry about having clients at the agency—they were assigned to me from a long waiting list. If they didn't show up, I often felt relief—I had time to do paperwork, get a cup of coffee, or shop online. But now, if clients didn't show up, I didn't get paid; if they didn't come back, it was because I didn't do a good job; if I didn't do a good job, word would get out, and I wouldn't get referrals. Down the rabbit hole I went with my fretting, and I had to work hard to pull myself back, say to myself that I was competent, that I would probably be older than anyone I would be seeing. Despite what my irrational brain was telling me, I wasn't that ten-year-old in the school play at risk of screwing up his lines.

I was surprised by all this angst, but it's understandable. Establishing a private practice involves building something on your own without the support you had before. There is the rational worry about how it will turn out. Expect this worry, and prep yourself for those bad days when you may need to talk yourself down.

Have a Vision

Tell me your vision of your ideal private practice. What would it look like in one, five, or ten years? Tell me about the office environment. Who would be your ideal client? Are there specific problems, clinical skills, and approaches you want to focus and build a reputation on? What type of work don't you want to do? How many hours a week do you want to work? Would you be working evenings or weekends? How much money do you want to make? What would an average day look like?

You're starting a new journey in your work life. Like road trips, sometimes the initial impetus is a restlessness—a need to get out of Dodge, to break away from agency life. But once you're under way, you want to set a course, and there's no better place to start than with the ideal. You want to avoid what I call precompromising, where you water down your vision before you even begin because of practicalities—you probably won't be able to do this; you can't afford that. If you start with this diluted vision, it's likely to become more and more diluted as real issues take hold. In a few years, your life is okay—not bad, but just okay. By starting with a bold and clear vision, you'll feel empowered. By keeping your eyes on your prize, your motivation will carry you forward on those days when you're wondering what you got yourself into.

Wade or Jump?

One way of reducing the pressure and worry is to wade into your private practice rather than diving off the high board. Many folks wade in by starting a side practice—a couple of nights a week after work, maybe a Saturday—seeing a few clients, negotiating with their employer, and cutting back from full time. I did consider having a side practice earlier in my career, but I bailed at the last minute. I realized that working a job and a half was too much; I was already burned out a lot of the time, and I didn't want to wind up having to wear a name tag for my wife and kids to know who I was. But this wading approach makes for an easier transition for some folks—you get to test the waters and not have to sweat income and can gradually make the break.

Just as you want to know the depth of the water before you sail off the high diving board, you want to know what to expect if you jump into your practice. Before I transitioned into private practice, I asked a couple of practitioners in my community about their experience: One said you needed to make twice the money you made at an agency to cover your overhead; the other said that it probably takes about six to nine months to get a full caseload; both were right. With this advice in mind, I not only crunched the numbers but also lined up some training gigs. You may want to do the same—have realistic expectations, find part-time work at a different agency or do supervision, say, at your former one, or simply get a part-time job in retail. Having a plan will give you a sense of control and reduce your anxiety.

Group or Solo?

Joining a group practice has several obvious advantages: You're making a transition from organization to organization, which is less mentally jarring; like your past organization, an infrastructure is in place—office space, billing systems, communication systems, and so on. You probably have a referral source—often, some intake system links potential clients with clinicians with particular specialties or openings. And you're not isolated: Even if it feels like you are passing in the night at times, there are colleagues around that you can chat with in the break room or get advice or even supervision from. All good.

Depending on the practice culture, the downside is that the group practice will likely include some of what you didn't like at your past agency. Yes, you're more independent—sharing space but doing your own thing—and there's an absence of hierarchy, but you still may be expected to attend weekly staff meetings or help cover for colleagues on vacation. You may not mind these extra responsibilities or feel that they waste your time. Finally, a group practice can also be more expensive than a solo practice. Many group practices are run like medical group practices, where you pay a set percentage of your monthly income rather than pay for your actual individual expenses. This is great when you're having a slow month but not so much when you're busy.

Just as beginning clinicians often stay at their first jobs for a few years to get their sea legs and then go into another setting or private practice, many who start in a group practice stay for a few years and then move on. Once they've built up a steady client load and a solid reputation, they go solo or start their own group practices.

Like wading versus jumping, if you decide to go solo from the start, either because there are no group practices near you or because going solo better suits your vision and personality, you again want to anticipate the downsides. If you're worried, for example, about the isolation, look for office space in a building with other professionals. (I attended a workshop once on starting your own practice, and the speaker suggested that you look for office space in a medical building—you'll have an opportunity to meet some doctors who can then be a referral source.) Or plan those twice-a-week lunches with other clinicians to talk shop and get support. Or connect with a supervisor who can offer you clinical feedback and reassurance and be that steady contact.

Getting the Word Out

Even though the group practice will help with advertising—it will put your bio on the practice website or place an announcement ad in the local paper—you also want to have your own website, and it is essential to have one if you are going solo. Having a website is how clients are most likely to find you; a website gives you the space to showcase yourself and your talents. Plenty of ready-made formats are available to peruse and can be tailored and styled to include the information you want, and they are also easy to create on your own. Look at the websites of your colleagues and see what you do or don't like.

One common mistake you want to avoid is describing yourself in terms that are too general: "I offer caring support to help you reach your potential in a safe environment." While this statement may convey an empathic tone, potential clients aren't generally looking for tone. They're looking for help with a particular problem—my anxiety, my relationship, my out-of-control child—that's the driver. Next, they want to know if you take their insurance. After that, they may want to know about your approach. Here you should include a profile statement about your clinical theory—long term versus short term, psychodynamic versus CBT. Many potential clients have been in therapy before, and even those who haven't know at least what they don't want—less or more focus on insight, less or more exploring the past, less or more problem solving. Finally, they look at your qualifications and expertise—your years of experience and track record.

Put all this information on your website—the problem areas you are most comfortable with or want to specialize in; what types of insurance you take; a clear statement of your approach—the psychodynamic versus the CBT. Build up your résumé—your years of experience, names of articles you have written, and programs you've started. Including these details is not bragging but selling yourself and, like it or not, promoting yourself is part of building a practice.

You also need to hit the streets. Find out if there is a monthly meeting of area family doctors and ask if you can give them a five-minute introduction to your practice. Volunteer at the local free clinic, where you can help patients with mental health issues and get to know the doctors who work there. Offer to do a free two-hour training on anxiety at the local nursing home. Give a talk at the monthly Rotary or Optimist Club meeting on stress and business management, motivation, or how to help children deal with trauma. Put yourself out there; see what sticks. People like to refer others to people they know.

Finally, join therapist directory sites. In the days before the internet, finding a therapist was often a clandestine process—quietly asking a coworker in the break room whether she knows of anyone who did couple therapy or asking your family doctor for a referral for depression. All that has changed. I estimate that about 70% of folks who contact me have found me by trolling through the internet and therapy directories. Get on them—have a good profile, include a picture of yourself, list your availability and the insurances you take.

Decide What You Are Willing to Do Yourself

Back to vision: Do you want to do your billing? Do you want someone to schedule your appointments? Do you want to clean your own bathrooms or hire a cleaning service? Again, paying other people to do these chores is the attraction of being in a group practice. But if you are working solo, figure out what you are willing to learn and do versus what will save you time and enable you to see more clients and not get burned out. Step back, think big picture. You are no longer a clinician but an entrepreneur running your own business.

Although there's both an emotional and practical learning curve to master as you move through this transition, it can also be a wonderful, empowering experience. Think big in terms of where you want to be; think small in terms of creating systems and routines that effectively and efficiently enable you to run your everyday new life. Most of all, damp down that self-criticism and have realistic expectations so you can realize that vision that you initially sought.

CHAPTER 51

Reflections

Looking Back at a Career

Looking back on it, the process seems pretty medieval now. A couple of months before finishing grad school, I started looking for a job and decided to focus on Atlanta. But there was no such thing as the internet; I didn't have access to the Atlanta newspapers. So, I had to go down to my public library, search the stacks, find the shelf full of Yellow Pages from major cities, and look up the phone numbers of mental health agencies in Atlanta. I then cold-called several, asking if they had openings. One agency finally said yes, and I was invited to come in for an interview. So I cut class, put on The Suit, and drove three hours.

The interview turned out to be a group interview, with five of us in the room sitting in a row like contestants in a spelling bee. Across from us sat three interviewers. One of them would ask us a question—about our experience, our clinical approach—which we then, in turn, answered. It was a bit bizarre; it had a game show vibe, with each of us jockeying to sound more intelligent, passionate, and creative than the others. Apparently, I didn't because I didn't get the job.

But I did get an interview, not in Atlanta but up the street from my school in Columbia, South Carolina. I was offered a job at Family Service Center, the oldest family services agency in continuous practice in the country, without doing much—no group interview, no questions about my clinical experience. The position came with a whopping annual salary of $8,000. (No, a loaf of bread didn't cost 25¢, but I did get a $200 raise the following year.) But I was on my way. I did home visits; saw individuals and families in the office; smoked a pipe in sessions (before anyone knew or cared about second-hand smoke) to fill silences, looked more professional and Freudian; and drank coffee all day. It's surprising that anything I said made sense. In two years, I supervised new hires; in three, I published my first journal article; in four, I was the Coordinator of Clinical Services. It was a small agency, with a staff of around 20, five of whom did therapy. I liked the family feel that it had. And being the only child I am, I was comfortable with the junior parent, rising-star role that I seemed to be in. After nine years I left, not because of the job but because I wanted to move to Virginia to be closer to family.

I rode into my new town all cocky, filled with a title, all that experience, and even more published articles under my belt. Six months later, I was depressed. No job. I had interviewed for only one position, and came in second out of 350 applicants. There were only a couple of places to work, and maybe I was overqualified or too cocky, who knows. I stayed at home with my kids, wallpapered my living room at 3:00 in the morning, and pumped iron while watching *Sesame Street* with my three-year-old daughter, thinking that moving was the stupidest thing I had ever done.

But then I started coming out of it. I started writing—a book that was never published, magazine articles that were. Finally, after a year and a half, I was offered a job doing kid work at the local mental health center. So impressed or desperate were they that they said I could work part time or full time, my pick. I chose part time, 24 hours a week. My son was a teen, and perhaps overcompensating for my father, who had always worked two jobs and never seemed to be around, I decided I wanted to spend time with my kids before they were gone.

Looking back on it, that year-plus of unemployment was difficult but pivotal. By not working, I slowed down, came to appreciate being a dad and a husband, and was able to start a separate career as a writer. If I had gotten that job right when I hit town, I probably would have fallen into a 40-hour-work-toward-retirement lifestyle and maybe never developed that writer part of me.

I eventually included more supervision in the job mix. I continued to write—magazine articles, an advice column for a national high-school magazine, a book on my supervision model, and articles for *Psychotherapy Networker.* It was a good mix, and I did it for twelve years. I wrote my first family therapy book, which led to other invitations and books. I was in my 40s or early 50s.

And my midlife crisis hit. My son was launched, my daughter was nearing graduation from high school, and I had the urge for something different, for . . . power. I applied for and got a job as Director of Child and Family Services at the same mental health center. We increased staff from fifteen to 50. I started several new programs, and I continued to write. I held this job for eight years, but then the worrying about budgets and hiring and all that goes with bureaucracies got to me. It was time for another change, and I decided to enter private practice.

Another "What was I thinking?" situation loomed up on many days. But I was better prepared than when I first moved to Virginia. Because of my street cred from books and articles, I got teaching gigs, traveling three days a week, twice a month to do day-long workshops on supervision, family and couple therapy, and brief therapy, which were exhausting but also fulfilling. My clinical work fed my writing and teaching, just as my teaching and writing fueled my clinical work. Having now lived through a pandemic, the workshops these days are remote, and because I'm getting older and losing some stamina, working remotely suits me fine.

And what did I learn from this arc of a career? I'm grateful for the opportunities that I stumbled upon, that were forced on me, and that I chose. I'm grateful that I found, or my life found, a way to let me use different aspects of me and my creativity, that I didn't get stuck in a box, that I had time to put my feet up on my desk and think big thoughts. I have no regrets and much to be thankful for, and that's about as good as it gets.

So, what do you want to be as you grow up? What talents and passions and nuggets of creativity in you do you want to mine? What are your priorities? What risks are you willing to take? What impact do you want to make on the lives of those around you? What do you want to be remembered for?

PART V

YOU

We started the book with you, and now we're back to you. In this last part, we're moving away from all our talk about clinical techniques, career arcs, work, and workplaces and returning to the you in your life. Some questions, some exercises, and hopefully some food for thought.

CHAPTER 52

Are You a Builder or a Discoverer?

Even if we can't fully articulate it, we each have a view of and relationship with our lives, specifically how we go about thinking about what we are to do with this stretch of time before us. We can break it down, I think, into two major approaches—that of builders and that of discoverers.

Builders

As the chapter title implies, builders build, with all that the word connotes. Life is about creating something, something tangible. You start with little or nothing, but you plan and assemble and . . . build. In my view, America is very builder oriented. You have roughly 40 years between 20 and 65 to make something of yourself. Ready, set, go!

Builders usually have clear objectives and a concrete sense of where they want to be at the finish line. Make law partner or be a judge. Start a business and reap the rewards of something grand. Or maybe not be work oriented, but be just as focused and driven—have three kids who will all turn out to be successful in their own way, a good home, and a contented life. Building is about plotting the course—finding the right partner, seizing those windows of opportunity, making good choices.

Builders can feel good when things are all falling into place, and when they don't, they are seen as challenges to be managed along the way. Builders can get excited about what's on the horizon but at times can also be myopic, seeing only what is three feet in front of them and little else. They can be self-critical, and some would say dangerously so caught up in running their lives that they're not living them.

As they near midlife or grow older, builders may realize that they may not accomplish what they set out to do, or that with their narrow focus, they have left too much of themselves out of the equation and have become one-dimensional. There may be resentment and regret that much of it was for naught. They are in danger of becoming depressed or, even if they were successful, crashing once the gold ring is won.

Discoverers

If life for the builders is a bit of the forced march with a blueprint in hand, for discoverers, it is more of a stroll along a path. Discoverers have goals, a direction they follow at the start, but they are not averse to exploring side roads and are curious about what may lie around the next corner. As with builders, the name says it all—life is to be discovered, the clear course is not always clear, and the obstacles along the path are challenges to confront or signs that there may be a better route. Failure isn't about self-criticism, but life telling you that this path isn't the one for you; it's time to try another.

While builders measure success in accomplishing their goals, discoverers measure their success in the accumulation of experiences, often in the good-enough life. But just as builders may feel a bit of panic as they near midlife or grow older and worry that their dreams will never be fulfilled, discoverers can panic and fear that they have drifted a bit too much, that the stroll perhaps should have been more of a determined march, that they don't have much to show for their travels as they near the finish line, that like the builders they've somehow not used the time well enough.

Going to the Other Side

Both builders and discoverers may decide at midlife to switch gears and adopt the other's perspective. Builders may slow down to smell the roses. They may go back down the road and gather up the parts of themselves that got left behind. They may allow curiosity and wants to replace shoulds and agendas.

Likewise, discoverers may realize they have little time left to get things done. Now at 45, they are talking about changing careers; the happy-to-be-a-line-worker now goes for the management job that they pooh-poohed for years; the stay-at-home mom decides she wants to go to law school. They hustle because they want to build something that can be a solid measure of their lives.

The Middle Ground

This is the space or the happy medium between these two perspectives. Having the blueprints and clear vision of the builder, but also keeping your ear close to the ground of yourself. Marching ahead, but periodically stopping to survey the terrain, see if the path is still the path you want to follow. Being curious, but not letting your curiosity take you too far astray into the weeds and away from your sense of purpose and values.

What side do you lean toward? Are there any adjustments, any course corrections, you need to make right now?

CHAPTER 53

Creating a Balanced Life

One of the challenges of this work is practicing what you preach. You talk to clients all day about the importance of self-care but, like them, you too can push this topic to the side. Here's my list of self-care tips—feel free to add your own.

Learn to Say No

We've talked about this several times, and we're talking about it again because, as caregivers, it's often difficult to do, and if you don't—you have no or too flaccid boundaries—you'll get drained and anxious.

Time to practice setting limits—turning off the phone or checking voice mail or emails twice a day, not 20; letting potential clients know you have a waiting list that you're happy to put them on; not automatically squeezing in that Friday afternoon appointment because the client is breathing heavily on the phone. Get your rational brain back online and decide if your worry is reasonable. If not, be bold. Say, in a therapeutic way, too bad. Yes, you will feel guilty and worry; do it anyway—this is about getting tough, saving yourself now so you can help others over the long haul.

Stop "Therapizing" Your Friends and Family

This is well known in the medical profession: New doctors see a patient with or learn about, say, tuberculosis, and now their mom's cough is viewed with suspicion, or their back pain isn't a strain from exercise but the beginning of kidney disease. You can easily fall into the same trap—seeing mental health problems springing up everywhere—your quiet brother is really depressed; your partner's procrastination means he has ADHD, your friend who checks that his door is locked three times before going to bed obviously is obsessive–compulsive and needs medication. And so, you intervene—talk about depression while your brother is grilling steaks; tell your partner how her pattern of putting things off indicates some executive functioning issues; you coach your friend about checking the door two times instead of three and give him the name of a psychiatrist that you know.

Time to learn to turn off that *on-duty* light. This tendency to keep it on is understandable because you're looking at the world through a new lens. But don't let your job and clinical perspective become your world. You are more than a therapist; it's okay to go off-duty and just be a person.

Have Many Baskets

There are folks who can't wait to retire after 30 years on the job. They do home projects for a few months but then run out of projects, play golf four times a week, and it gets old. Or they volunteer to serve on a nonprofit board for a year, but then get bored. They crash; they get depressed. They're missing and grieving their old life and the identity and purpose it provided. They put all their eggs into their work basket, and now the basket has been tipped over and they are scrambling and hurting.

Instead, you want to have multiple baskets and develop them early—your work basket, your family or children basket, your hobby or passion basket—painting, studying the Civil War, knitting—whatever. As financial advisors say, you need to stay diversified, so if something goes down in one sector, it's compensated for by something else. Don't put all of you into your job.

Fix Your Personal Problems

You have untreated ADHD; your intimate relationship has grown less and less intimate each year; you smoke pot too much and are haunted by childhood wounds or loneliness. This stuff can bleed into your clinical work, creating those deadly countertransferences, those subtle biases, those blind spots that cause you to over- or underreact with clients. But over the long haul, unresolved personal problems drain your creativity, potential, and enjoyment of life. It's time for the healer to heal himself.

Build Stress Reduction into Your Everyday Life

You tell your clients to try to reduce stress all the time, but for some reason, you don't see to it—the exercise, meditation, good diet, mini-vacations. If you need to be guilted into reducing stress, realize that you want to be a good role model for your clients or your kids.

Daydream

Covey's not urgent/not important tasks *are* important—putting your feet up on your desk, brainstorming, and daydreaming. Make room in your life for inspiration, out-of-the-box thinking, big thoughts. Doing so requires you to slow down and listen to your inner self, to discover and nurture those seeds of change, those quiet voices.

What's the one thing you need to stop doing that would make the biggest difference? What do you need to start doing that would make the biggest difference?

Can you stop—or start . . . today?

CHAPTER 54

Getting Closure

Writing to Heal Old Wounds

Unfortunately, like a lot of guys, Sam didn't grieve much when his dad died. He had to take care of his mom, handle the funeral and estate, and at the time, essentially became the good soldier, burying most of his emotions. But, years later, this unresolved grief over his father is now taking its toll—he's constantly anxious and irritable.

Terry was fired from her job, unfairly she felt. Although other staff members were struggling with the same problems she was, she felt that her boss was singling her out. Months later, she is resentful and depressed.

What Sam and Terry have in common is a lack of closure. Sam never went through the grief process around the loss of his dad; Terry never got a chance to confront her boss and get things off her chest. These unresolved emotions and unexpressed feelings can be like an undertow in your life that keeps you from emotionally and behaviorally moving forward.

Sam and Terry are not alone—I, maybe you, maybe most of us all have something, some baggage from the past we still carry that weighs us down and slows our forward progress. It haunts us, keeps pulling us into the past, colors our present, and obscures our future. For some of us, like Sam, it is about grief and loss and relationships; for others, it's about what's not been said but needs to be said; and for still others, it's about stopping the internal battle with some chronic emotional or physical problem—addiction, trauma, depression. It's about changing the story by changing the story.

If lack of closure is something you're struggling with, here is a simple yet powerful exercise to try.

Write three letters. Find a quiet place and a time when you are not rushed to do this exercise. You literally want to write the letters using pen and paper, not a computer or mobile phone, and write in a stream of consciousness. Rather than approaching the exercise as you would a high school essay, you want to let your mind go and write down your flowing thoughts—such as "I don't know where to start," "This is stupid." Try to do this all in one sitting.

Next, consider whatever you need to get closure on or to be reconciled with. Imagine what this problem or person looks like.

Now imagine it or the person sitting in the chair next to you; it or the person is only there for one hour, and then is gone, never coming back.

Letter 1

Write down everything you wished you had said or want to say now. Sam may talk about how much he loved his dad, express his anger over something that happened when he was young, or describe his memories of a family trip when he was four. Terry may write about her anger and the unfairness or what she misses most about her job. What is it you need to get off your chest and say most? Again, let your mind guide you. Don't worry about grammar and punctuation. Write. Take your time, and see what emerges.

After about ten, fifteen, or 20 minutes, you may hit a wall and run out of things to say. Take a couple of deep breaths. See if you get a second wind. If so, start writing again. At some point, you'll have a sense of being done.

Letter 2

Now, if this other person were to get Letter 1 or to hear what you said, what do you think that person would say back? Write the person's response down. If, for example, Sam's dad was a bit crusty and closed, he might say something short and sweet like, "Thanks, Sam, got your letter; I love you too." Terry's boss may sound defensive—"Our policy has always been . . . " This letter could be optional if the person was open and your relationship was good.

Letter 3

This one is probably the most important. This time write down all you would *want* the person or the problem to say back after reading your first letter. Sam's dad may talk not only about how proud he is of Sam, but also about his own regrets as a dad—that he wasn't available or that he realized he was overbearing at times—or his own memories of their time together or his own struggles as an adult. Terry's boss may say she did realize that she was singling Terry out, apologize, and then explain why—that she was threatened by her skills or has always had a difficult time with assertive women, which really has nothing to do with Terry.

Let your imagination go, settle down deep into your feelings, and see what comes to the surface. What you hear (and write down in Letter 3) may be not only surprising but healing as well.

When you've completed the three letters, step away from them for a short time, but then reread them aloud to yourself or ideally to someone close to you who can just listen. The process of rereading the letters may stir up some strong and sad emotions. Again, leave yourself plenty of time to do this.

This exercise can be emotionally powerful on a couple of levels. Obviously, you are completing the circle by saying what you couldn't say and hearing what you didn't hear but needed to. But because all losses are connected emotionally, you may be healing older and still deeper wounds of the past at the same time (you may find yourself shifting gears as you write and find yourself thinking about or talking to someone else once you start). That's fine—just let it out.

Again, take your time, don't hold back.

It's time to put the past to rest.

CHAPTER 55

Reflections

My Big Day in Court

Sometimes you don't get a chance to run toward what you fear; instead, it comes to you. A few months after grad school, I was assigned a custody case that required that I do a home study: interviewing the mother and her children in the home to assess their relationship and size up the environment. And so out I went. The house looked like a shack from the dirt road it sat on, but the inside, I noticed, was squeaky clean—check. A gaggle of preschoolers scattered about the house, but the mother managed to scoop them up and corral them into a circle of sorts, with the oldest girl helping contain the younger ones—another check. And the mother talked about her worries for the children, and how her husband had left, but she was doing the best she could. She seemed nice; she seemed sincere. Okay, assessment done, case closed—a wrap.

I imagined that I would maybe have to type up my notes or have a phone conversation with the social services worker about my impressions at some point. But no! Instead, I received a subpoena to testify in court. I had never been in a courtroom in my life, let alone having to testify. So I donned The Suit, showed up, and was called to the stand by one of the attorneys.

"So before you give your expert testimony, could you please tell the court about your professional experience?"

I'm already stumped and scrambling. What professional background? I had an office with my name on the door. The attorney, seeing my flustered hesitation, came to my aid. I realized he was my good guy in the case.

"So, can you tell the court where you went to graduate school?" I mumbled an answer. "And I see here you are a member of . . . the National Association of Social Workers . . . ?" I nodded. To me, this felt like one step above "And can you testify to the court that you can read and write your own name?"

At this point, the other attorney, the bad one, stood up and challenged my being sworn in as an expert witness. Totally understandable, I thought—what the heck was I doing there; no legal rocket science needed to make that call. And the judge, in his judicial voice and with the slamming of the gavel, called for an adjournment to discuss . . . me. I was expelled from the courtroom. I could only imagine what they were saying about me behind my back as I sat on a bench in the hall. And then I got called back in, and was somehow back on the witness stand, and the nice attorney asked me about my home visit.

I did the best I could while feeling like a ten-year-old. I sat up straight; I tried not to croak my voice as the good attorney lobbed me simple questions—was the house clean, were the kids dressed—and I tried to turn my "she was a nice lady" assessment into the best professional jargon I could think of at the time, though I have no recollection of what I said. And then it was done—seconds, minutes, hours later—I don't remember. I left the courtroom shell-shocked, the way you feel after a car accident or after receiving unexpected bad news, not knowing or caring what actually was the outcome of the case.

I wandered back to my office, slump-shouldered and weary like a soldier after miraculously surviving some horrendous battle. And like that shell-shocked trauma victim, I felt the need to get out my story, to process what had just happened. It was the end of the day. I wandered into my supervisor's office and, not only was she free, but also a few of the older staff magically seemed to gather. As I reenacted all the gory details of my experience (the same way a young teen may play out for his parents the movie he had just seen), my kind audience jumped in with their own stories of their first courtroom experiences—the same shell shock, the same feeling of being stupid and overwhelmed. And when they looked back on the experience, their deciding that it eventually made a good story. That old adage: Comedy = Tragedy + Time.

It turned out they were right.

CHAPTER 56

Run toward What You Fear

We talked about the three ways of coping with anxiety—approach, avoid, bind. Piling onto this topic a bit more is this notion of running toward what you fear. Approaching is a great antidote to anything in your life that creates anxiety. This idea is the basis of exposure therapy—sitting next to that snake in the cage when you have a phobia of snakes; washing your hands four times instead of five when you're anxious about germs. And also approaching more extreme challenges: Climb up that 20-foot pole, then jump over to the next one; survive in the woods by yourself for a month with a knife and a flint.

Approaching such difficult and frightening situations runs counter to what your anxious brain is telling you: "If you don't want to feel anxious, just listen to me: Pull in, be cautious, don't do." Don't go to that party where you don't know anyone; don't confront your partner about his drinking; don't go back into that Walmart where you had your panic attack. Avoid, keep your world small, don't do, and you'll feel safe.

Although you can't undo those old anxious circuits in your brain, you can keep them from firing and getting stronger by creating new ones. And you do this by pushing through rather than pushing away, expanding your comfort zone, and desensitizing yourself to the feeling of anxiety. And when you come out on the other side and find out that what you thought was going to happen didn't, your view of the world as a scary place begins to change. Your self-confidence grows and your self-image improves. Approaching is a good way to run your life.

It is also a good way to conduct your work. Undoubtedly there are a bunch of things that you feel anxious about. They may involve seeing certain types of clients—aggressive men, for example—or dealing with problems that you are clueless about handling—kids with ADHD, narcissistic personalities, or couple therapy. Or attempting new skills—doing play therapy—navigating outside-the-normal-box situations—testifying in court, serving on an interagency committee. Everyone's got something, but the point is that rather than waking up at 3:00 in the morning worrying about some problem or doing your best to avoid it, go proactive and run toward what you're afraid of. Talk to your supervisor about getting training or coaching in play therapy, sit in on a couple of therapy sessions with a colleague, visit a courtroom and observe how testimony is delivered, and get some tips on managing kids with ADHD in a session. You'll still have to take that leap at some point—jump to the next pole—but at least you'll be a bit better prepared and a bit less anxious. And if you pat yourself on the back for both taking the initiative in the first place and making the leap regardless of how it turns out, you've got it made.

What are you afraid of most? What do you need to learn to run toward?

CHAPTER 57

Your Life as a Movie

Here's a short exercise to help you check in on the state of your life. Pretend you are a screenwriter or a novelist creating the outline for a new movie or novel based on you and your life. Ask yourself these seven questions to get you started.

1. How Would You Describe Yourself, the Main Character?

These descriptions generally show up in the first few pages of novels: Sara has green eyes; Makeem can't help focusing on details; Juan is fascinated by butterflies. Think in terms of both your physical and personality traits. Notice what traits you think of first on both counts.

But then drill down: Is there anything else about you that you consider important parts of your physical self or personality that are often overlooked by others and yourself? How might others describe you?

Our views of ourselves are often based on how others see us, or we adopt a too-simple view of ourselves. What is the gap between how you see yourself and how others see you? What do you need to do to close that gap? Do you need or want to bring other, often overlooked traits more to the forefront of your life to expand your self-image?

2. What Other Characters Play an Essential Role in This Story?

Except for novels like *War and Peace* perhaps, most stories don't have hundreds of characters but have a few important and often pivotal ones—best friends, parents, mentors, enemies, frenemies.

Building your life also includes appreciating those people who have helped you build your life. When you step back, who has or is now pivotal for you in your life—who are the steady influences, supports, or sources of frustrations or challenges? How do you possibly need to change these relationships?

3. What Is the Core Conflict?

Every story has some conflict, and so does every life. It may be internal—the protagonist struggling with the trauma of the past or an addiction—Gollum in *The Lord of the Rings* with his light and dark sides—or in coming-of-age movies about who the main character wants to be. Or maybe it is about external conflicts with others—Sherlock Holmes had his Moriarity; Batman, the Joker—or with the outside world—the whistle-blower and her values versus the organization.

When you look back, is there a core conflict for you—internally, externally, or both—that has lingered, a thread that runs through the fabric of your life that you even now continue to struggle with?

4. What Is the Main Character's Number-One Goal, Her Quest?

Win the war, save the family, get off the island, make a million dollars, find Nemo. This goal is about having a purpose and focus—maybe it's something right now, and immediate, but often it's something larger and longer—the powerful psychological driver that impacts everything the character tries to do.

Step back: What is your number-one goal, your quest that shapes who you are and want to be?

5. What Obstacles Get in the Way of Reaching Your Goal(s)?

Sleeping Beauty's prince needs to get through the forest of thorns; Indiana Jones needs to decode the riddles; Frodo needs to get to Mount Doom and destroy the ring. What are the obstacles that challenge you in your quest? They may be internal—that you are impulsive or perfectionistic or lack confidence or have a temper—or external—that you lack money or emotional support.

What are the one or two obstacles that seem to get in your way of succeeding?

6. What Do You Need to Overcome These Obstacles?

Frodo had Sam and Gandalf, Sherlock Holmes had Dr. Watson, Captain Kirk had Bones and Spock. But for others, succeeding requires learning about determination or commitment, about being able to walk away, about facing that addiction or anxiety, about learning to appreciate what you have, or about thinking outside the box.

What is it you need most within and outside you to succeed?

7. How Do You Want the Story to End?

You return the ring, you kiss the princess, you get the Olympic gold medal. Or you reconcile with your family, become a better parent, or develop the self-confidence that allows you to believe in yourself and reach your goals.

This part of your story is important: You have control over the ending because you and only you can make decisions and have choices about where your life will go and what will happen to our hero, even if those choices seem at times so limited.

Envision your future, the ending that you want to create. What will it be?

CHAPTER 58

What's Your Relationship with Your Life?

How do you think about your "life"?

For many people, life becomes a montage of both good and bad scenes from the past—a combination of emotions, photo images, or some chronological march through the highlights of past years. Others measure their lives in increments, like black lines on a ruler—the last couple of years have been good; the ones before pretty rough.

But what if you thought of your life as something more present, more active, and not as marks on a ruler or a portfolio of memories about where you've been but more like a companion, separate from you, but one that always walks beside you through this thing called life.

Can you imagine this? Close your eyes. Imagine your life as a person emerging from the edge of a wood, from out of a fog. Take your time. Now start a conversation with this person. What's your relationship with your life like?

If You Were Roommates, How Would You Describe Your Relationship with Your Life?

We're good-enough friends: We check in with each other and talk about how we're doing, make sure we are both doing okay. Or we're best friends: We're emotionally close; we share confidences; we feel like we are a team and have each other's backs. Or no, we don't get along at all: We're constantly criticizing each other; I feel she's always working against me, is always unhappy about something, and there's constant tension. Or I try never to think about her at all.

Can you trust and lean into your life or not, because there is always blaming, criticism, or avoidance?

If Your Life is a Close Friend, Then Who Tends to Take the Lead?

This conversation is about whether you see your life as one that you build—as we discussed earlier—where you take the lead, set goals, and march forward, and your life follows along behind you. Or do you see your life as one that you discover—where your life is in the lead and you trust its ability to guide and show the way, trust that you will always wind up where you need to be, and trust those small voices or instincts and stay open to whatever path seems to open? Or is it some combination of building and discovering: At times, you are determined, focused, and proactive, but at other times, you are curious or uncertain and willing to see what evolves?

Do You Like the Path That You and Your Life Are Currently Following?

Are you both going in the direction you want to go in, or are you following a path because it is one that you traveled before, the only path your life knows? Do you struggle over what fork in the road to take? Is there a path less traveled that you want to explore?

Can You and Your Life Work it Out if There is a Conflict?

This conversation is about the conflicts inside us—between the wants and shoulds, taking this path or another one, about following your heart or your mind. Can you hear and weigh both sides, or is your life more of a bully ceaselessly pressing you to do what it wants?

How Do You Want to Change Your Relationship with Your Life?

What would you want to change about your relationship with your life? Stop with the criticism and be more gentle; let's give each other the support and courage needed to take another road; take the lead, have your life trust you and simply follow behind for a while.

You and your life, a relationship like any other. What do you appreciate? What do you want to change?

CHAPTER 59

How to Be Wise

If building and discovering are about how to think about your life, how to be wise is about simply how to be. We associate wisdom with old age, the accumulation of knowledge that comes from encountering life's trials and tribulations, but obviously, not everyone who is old is wise. Wisdom is not just the result of sorting through a lap full of experience. It is also a product of learning fundamental ways of viewing your life and the world around you as you move forward.

Here is a list of wisdom characteristics and the steps to its achievement. As you consider them, think about the wise people that you know.

Be Honest with Yourself

You undoubtedly know from working with clients how this simple statement is more complicated than it seems. On one level, it is about self-awareness: realizing and being able to define your emotions; knowing your values and priorities—what is important in life and what it means to be a "good" person; knowing what you want—being able to use your gut reactions and instincts, rather than just the rules in your head, to let you know what you need.

But at another level, being honest is about having the courage to recognize your faults, honor your struggles, admit mistakes, and take full responsibility for your decisions and actions, rather than blaming others or the circumstances.

Be Honest with Others

Self-honesty is an important first step because if you can't be honest with yourself, you can't ever reveal and articulate what is truly you. But even if you get through that hurdle, there's another one in which you may get stuck. Even though you know what you think and believe, you may feel vulnerable, unsafe, fearful, and worried about others' reactions. You sugarcoat your complaints about the job, bite your tongue, and don't tell your partner what you are upset about or want changed. You hold back.

The danger in not being honest with others is that you begin to feel isolated because no one really knows you; the problems that bother you back up over time, leading to explosions or depression. The antidote is to override your old coping style and develop the courage to step up even though your instincts say to step down.

Focus on the Process Rather Than on the Outcome

While the first two suggestions are about having an honest dialogue with yourself and others, this step is more about your behaviors and how you approach tasks. The outcome is obviously about the result, the goal, the end. We tend to think of process as merely the means to reaching that end.

We've talked a lot about the importance of process in this book, and those folks we consider wise have somehow learned that lesson—making process, rather than outcome, an end in itself. Those who focus only on the outcome often feel frustrated or driven; they lose sight of the everyday pleasures of running their lives; they measure their happiness by measuring themselves against others and, by doing so, give up their power. But by focusing your attention on what you are doing, measuring your happiness by what unfolds, and letting go of your expectations of the results, you not only can stay in the present rather than in the future and close to your changing needs and, as the sages say, living in the only place that life is and that you can control.

Listen to the Changes in Yourself

But even if you focus on the process and the present, you still need to listen, to slow down enough to catch those subtle changes naturally evolving inside you. Those who do the forced march through life—as many of our clients do—those who push away their emotions or dreams or anger often fall into depression or emotional crisis.

Make time to periodically take stock of your life.

Learn from Mistakes

Older people, and particularly wise people, generally have an easier time living their lives. Looking back, I realize that my life is much easier now than when I was in my 20s and 30s, maybe even in my 40s. Why? Not because I have fewer problems, but because I've realized that life is a process of elimination. Over the years, I've learned enough lessons along the way—from how to change a water filter to how to talk to my children so that they feel supported and understood and to how to listen to and take care of myself—that the number of lessons left to learn has grown smaller.

Imbedded in all problems are lessons to learn. Once you learn the lesson that the problem is trying to teach—that you shouldn't rant at your boss or partner, that you need to check the oil in your car—the problem goes away. If you don't, the problem keeps coming up.

Where it is easy to get stuck is in never taking the time to sit back and reflect on the lesson that is embedded in that problem, your past experience. There's always a moral to the story. You undoubtedly see or will see clients whose hardships only confirm the same story: That others can't be trusted and are out to hurt you; that life is unfair. Or no, it's not others but you who victimize you—instead of blaming others, you blame yourself—that you're not good enough, that you deserve what you get.

Obviously, there are good reasons for holding on to these stories. But succeeding in life and being wise comes by learning from life and changing the story.

Have a Sense of Humor

Maybe humor is too strong a word here—we're not talking about doing stand-up. But what is applicable is what we mentioned before—the definition of comedy: tragedy plus time. What this translates into on your quest to be wise is an ability to step back, put what seem like big problems and events into perspective, and sort out your priorities so that not everything feels so important and overwhelming, to see a first-world problem as a first-world problem. It's also about realizing that what feels so important today, this month, and this year is likely to change over time—because of time itself, because of your accumulating wisdom.

This too shall pass; this will, at some point, make for an interesting story.

Be Kind to Others

Yes, this sounds like the platitude that everyone knows. But what is behind it is not only about how you treat others, but also how you see the world. Kindness comes from seeing you and others as connected in some way, that though we are different, we all are struggling in our own ways, and with this filter in place, you can be empathic. Without it, life is about competition, a hunger game where others can't be trusted, where it's every person for themselves. Sure, you may be the one to come out on top, but it comes at the cost of a life filled with anxiety, paranoia, and loneliness.

Find and Believe in Your Contribution to the World

If there is one takeaway from this book, it is this: Ask yourself these questions: What is your purpose? What difference do you hope to make by living your life, and how do you measure it? What can you do that no one else can do? What makes a good-enough life, and how do you decide? These are existential questions, not clinical ones. Step back, reflect, ask, and listen.

Okay, that's my list; you may find that you have others to add. The theme that runs through these suggestions is the notion that wisdom can be achieved from culling the best of life's experiences and learning from them; by keeping your hands on the steering wheel of your life; by being assertive, active, and clear-eyed; by periodically stepping back and seeing how well your outer life represents your inner one; by putting into place your own, and often hard-earned, values about how you treat yourself and others. It's not something that you achieve or not in later life, but is rather a way of living your life right now.

Ultimately, becoming wise is simply you becoming most fully you.

We've reached the end of our journey. I hope this guidebook has served its purpose—of helping you know what is ahead, what to see and what to avoid, what to make the most of in this journey called work, a career, a calling, and a life.

Thank you, as always, for taking me along.

References

Berg, M., & Maloney, D. (2003). *There is no road: Proverbs by Antonio Machado.* White Pines Press.

Bowen, M. (1993). *Family therapy in clinical practice.* Jason Aronson.

Brown, G. S. J., Lambert, M. J., Jones, E. R., & Minami, T. (2005). Identifying highly effective psychotherapists in a managed care environment. *American Journal of Managed Care, 11*(8), 513–520.

Covey, S. (2020). *The 7 habits of highly effective people.* Simon & Schuster.

Duhigg, C. (2014). *The power of habit.* Random House.

Gilbert, R. M. (1992). *Extraordinary relationships: A new way of thinking about human interactions.* Wiley.

Karpman, S. (1968). Fairy tales and script drama analysis. *Transactional Analysis Bulletin, 7*(26), 39–43.

Leichsenring, F., Rabung, S., & Leibing, E. (2004). The efficacy of short-term psychodynamic psychotherapy in specific psychiatric disorders: A meta-analysis. *Archives of General Psychiatry, 61*(12), 1208–1216.

Mueller, W., & Kell, B. (1972). *Coping with conflict: Supervising counselors and psychotherapists.* Appleton-Century-Crofts.

Taibbi, R. (2019). *Process-focused therapy: A guide for creating effective clinical outcomes.* Routledge.

Taibbi, R. (2022). *Doing family therapy: Craft and creativity in clinical practice* (4th ed.). Guilford Press.

Wang, L. (2019). *Psychiatrists have the highest suicide rate of any profession. It's time to do something about it.* https://medium.com/invisible-illness/psychiatrists-have-the-highest-suicide-rate-of-any-profession-its-time-to-do-something-about-it-7d63e2f2fe21.

Index